'This book is essential reading for women who are affected every month by the premenstrual syndrome.'

Here's Health

'. . . her book is comprehensive and above all practical.'

Successful Slimming

'Dr Caroline Shreeve brings hope for all sufferers from the premenstrual syndrome.'

Company

The Premenstrual Syndrome

This book is for the many thousands of women who, every month, find their lives affected by symptoms of premenstrual syndrome. Here, at last, is not only sympathy and understanding, but a wealth of practical advice, and also news of a natural, drug-free cure.

By the same author
DEPRESSION
DIVORCE
THE HEALING POWER OF HYPNOTISM
(with David Shreeve)

The Premenstrual Syndrome
The Curse that <u>Can</u> be Cured

by

Caroline Shreeve
M.D., B.S.(Lond.), L.R.C.P., M.R.C.S.(Eng.)

THORSONS PUBLISHERS LIMITED
Wellingborough, Northamptonshire

First published 1983
Sixth Impression 1986

British Library Cataloguing in Publication Data

Shreeve, Caroline Mozelle
  The premenstrual syndrome
  1. Premenstrual syndrome
  I. Title
  618.1'7206   RG165

  ISBN 0-7225-0829-8

Printed and bound in Great Britain

Dedication

This book is dedicated to my mother, Bertha Mary Pocock, who has weathered many changing attitudes to women over a period of eight decades yet retained her patience and her humour.

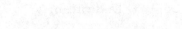

Contents

Introduction

Throughout the ages, many societies have held the belief that menstruating women are 'unclean'; other societies even consider them to be dangerous! In the majority of primitive tribes, women are held as taboo during their periods, while in some, superstition runs so rife with respect to the evil power of menstrual blood, that entire herds of cattle are expected to languish and die if they pass over ground upon which a drop of this noxious fluid has fallen. The women are obliged to conceal themselves from the sight of men, and even to avoid touching clothes, cooking vessels and sleeping mats belonging to their menfolk lest the latter should fall ill and waste away.

This attitude is not confined to one culture or even to one ethnic group: on the contary, evidence suggests that the feeling is widespread throughout the uncivilized world. In a number of Australian tribes, for example, a menstruating woman is severely scolded or beaten by her husband or nearest relative if she fails to warn approaching males of her condition. In other tribes of that continent the seclusion of menstruating women is even more rigid, and enforced by worse penalties than these – if, during her period, a woman of the Wakelbura tribe enters the encampment by the same route as the men, she may be put to death.

The Mohammedan scriptures have the following to say on the subject, in the Medinan chapters of the Koran:

> And they ask thee about menstruation. Say: It is harmful; so keep aloof from women during menstrual discharge and go not near them until they are clean. But when they have cleansed themselves, go in to them as Allah has commanded you. Surely Allah loves those who turn much to him, and he loves those who purify themselves.

The Bushmen of South Africa believe that a glance from a girl's eye, at the time when she should be kept in strict retirement, can fix men in whatever position they happen to occupy, with whatever they are holding in their hands, and change them into trees that are able to talk.

Some societies dread the onset of female puberty even more than the recurrent menstrual flow. Among the Zulus and some other African peoples, the girls themselves believe that the sun shining on their heads during the arrival of their first period, will wither them up into skeletons. This is why they hide away in the undergrowth with their blankets over their heads until the sun goes down, should the first signs of menstruation catch them unawares while they are working in the fields or gathering wood.

In New Ireland, in the United States (at least during the early part of this century), dread of a girl's pubertal development was such that pre-pubertal girls were confined to small cages for four or five years before, during and after the onset of puberty, kept in the dark and forbidden to set foot on the ground – at the end of which time they were led out to their marriage feasts.

The customs and beliefs of primitive tribes may seem, at first glance, no more than interesting, probably anachronistic, accounts more appropriate to an anthropological work than a book about the premenstrual syndrome. But take a closer look and there exist points of striking relevance to modern, civilized women in twentieth-century Western society – one which, while highly advanced in many respects, still clings unconsciously to a number of outdated beliefs springing from deep wells of fear, ignorance and superstition.

Certainly throughout the history of our society, menstruating women have not inspired the same kind of terror that has caused them within other societies to be socially ostracized and forcibly segregated. Had this been the case, then the course of our history may well have run quite differently. Boadicea might never have dealt the invading Romans a sharp rap over the knuckles had her period started just as she was about to sweep forth in her chariot to avenge the rape of her daughters – and she had been led away by female members of the Iceni tribe to a week of solitary confinement instead!

If Elizabeth I had been confined to her private chambers for seven days out of every twenty-eight that she reigned, would she have been so astute a stateswoman and so successful a queen? The answer is a definite 'no' – although the irreverent thought does spring to mind that she may well have been suffering from irrational anger or uncontrollable urges to violence due to the premenstrual syndrome when she signed the death warrant of Mary, Queen of Scots!

Again, the history of the nursing profession might have been a different story, had Florence Nightingale's job been interrupted every time her period arrived, as she strove to lay the foundation of the modern noble edifice and wrest the then menial job of caring for the sick from the hands of gin-sodden midwives and ignorant, if well-meaning, ladies bountiful.

The attitude of our own society to women's periods, and all that they entail, is reflected in the names that have been used to refer to that time of the month. Years ago, the name 'the curse' was coined, and became firmly established despite the changing fashions of popular speech, and I feel that the main reason for the durability of the term is its great appropriateness in two senses. Firstly, menstrual periods and their attendant premenstrual phase are a curse if managed badly or left untreated. Secondly, the religious connotation of *the,* rather than *a,* curse seems to substantiate the widely held belief that uncomfortable periods have devolved upon women as a direct result of misbehaviour in the Garden of Eden.

Eve, the archetypal mother, disobeyed God in long-lost Paradise and caused Adam to follow suit, for which she was punished by the original curse. In other words, and in practical, everyday terms, the first woman of the human race, according to our mythology, lost her claim to a perpetual life of contentment and ease, unvisited by old age and disease, and assumed the physical state that all subsequent human beings came to accept as inseparable from our mortal and tenuous existance. No longer immune from sickness and suffering, Eve no doubt was visited by her full share of monthly bleeding and pain and – as the premenstrual syndrome tends to grow worse as women grow older and bear several children – by the discomfort and emotional upheaval of this as well. This is what all women have experienced since then and what, for centuries, we have been expected to bear – rather along the lines of: 'the sins of the fathers shall be visited upon the children, even unto the final generation. . .'

Gibbon, the historian of the declining Roman empire, wrote these unforgettable words:

> The chaste severity of the fathers in whatever related to the commerce of the two sexes flowed from the same principle – their abhorrence of every enjoyment which might gratify the sensual and degrade the spiritual nature of man. It was their favourite opinion that, if Adam had preserved his obedience to the Creator, he would have lived forever in a state of virgin purity, and that some harmless mode of vegetation might have peopled Paradise with a race of innocent and immortal beings. The use of marriage was permitted only to his fallen posterity, as a necessary expedient to continue the human species, and as a restraint . . . Since desire was imputed as a crime, and marriage was tolerated as a defect, it was consistent with the same principles to consider a state of celibacy as the nearest approach to the divine perfection.

For thousands of years – up to and including decades of the present century – very little, if anything, was done to alleviate the unpleasant symptoms which the vast majority of women experience while they are menstruating, nor the whole complex (or syndrome) of problems, mental and physical, which effect far more women than is generally realized during the premenstrual phase of their cycle. This is partly accounted for by the fact that sex and the reproductive system were taboo conversational topics. Certainly the advent of sex education in schools and movements to establish equal rights for women, as well as a more liberal attitude towards sexual activity, have contributed to alerting the scientific and medical world to the subject of 'women's complaints'. To a certain extent, the earlier ignorance has been, or is being, rectified. As women become more aware of their own identities, so they develop body-consciousness and thereby an awareness of how their bodies work, and what these feel like when they are not working properly. Because women now talk openly to one another and to their doctors, the full range of menstrual problems has come to light.

This means that painful periods, with their cramps, excessive blood loss, fatigue, backache, listlessness, depression and weight gain, can all be dealt with satisfactorily. Only quite recently, though, has the premenstrual syndrome emerged as a major cause of women's emotional problems and physical ailments, and provided the explanation for many apparently disparate symptoms and complaints. To get an idea of just how recently, think back to what you were told about periods, and what to expect from them, when you were at school. If, like me, most of your schooling took place during the 1950s, (and especially if, like me, you were educated in a Convent boarding school), you were probably told nothing at all about periods by the teachers, and had to pick up what little knowledge you could from your mother or an elder sister if you were lucky, or from whispered 'secrets' in the cloakroom and surreptitious forays into the school library dictionary if you were not.

If your school days occurred during the 1960s, your biology lessons may have expanded upon the bare facts of the hormonal monthly cycle of the female mammal chosen for syllabus study, and included a few helpful details about periods in the human female as well. Social implications may have been touched upon, and perhaps some information volunteered about the production of pelvic and back pain by engorged pelvic blood vessels and contracting uterine muscle. Discussions with school friends would have been freer and more enlightened than a decade earlier and would probably have grappled with the eternal question of choosing internal or external sanitary protection.

If you were at school during the 1970s, discussions about sex, periods, pregnancy and related subjects would have been still more open. Sex education classes, as they came to be called, were fairly explicit in many schools and well-planned courses encouraged the open exchange of viewpoints between class and teacher, and between the pupils themselves. Books, slides and films explaining and describing many aspects of the subject were available, and the emphasis of concern tended to switch from choice of sanitary protection, and who had/had not yet started their periods, to the choice of contraceptive. In the cases of girls – and boys – who 'chanced' intercourse without protective measures, the topic of whether so-and-so might be pregnant became a common concern.

By this time, girls had become a great deal more sophisticated, in a limited sense, than those of the same age group a couple of decades earlier, and, at a superficial level, were more emotionally mature. It is now the norm for teenage girls to be relatively well informed on such topics as menstrual periods, sexual intercourse and pregnancy – at least in its early stages. Many are on the Pill – some for contraceptive purposes and the rest to correct irregular periods or severe period pain.

Most girls and young women nowadays know that uncomfortable periods can be remedied, and they seek their doctor's advice without embarrassment for persistent menstrual trouble. We have now reached the stage at which knowledge of the premenstrual syndrome – what it is, whether you are suffering from it, and what to do if you are – needs to be far more widely spread. A number of women remain unconvinced that periods produce symptoms requiring understanding and medical treatment, let alone accept the possibility that the premenstrual syndrome exists. Many such women, whom I have seen in surgery, are old enough to have lived through one or both World Wars, and therefore were probably at school during the second decade of the century. In the main, they have had hard, menial jobs during and since their teenage years, and tend to have come from a large family and to have had at least three children themselves. Personality characteristics include a high moral code, a diligent attitude to work, and, generally, fidelity to their husbands. They claim that 'the curse' is a lot of nonsense, and have little patience with women who complain of aches and pains during their periods.

Mary Weston was a fairly typical example of this kind of lady. Aged sixty-one, and the mother of several sons and daughters, she came to see me about her bunions and dropped arches. She worked as an office cleaner and had for years supported an indolent, boozy husband and the mongol son of one of her daughters who had 'got into trouble' shortly after leaving school. I offered her a week off work as her feet were in a sorry condition and she deserved a rest. She was quite offended! She replied that all she had come for was to get something to rub on her aching feet and not to be 'mollycoddled like young people are nowadays'. I was treating the errant daughter for menstrual trouble, so I suspected that it was Emily to whom she was referring. She mentioned her, and declared that she did not hold with women and girls taking time off work just because it was their time of the month – despite the fact that Emily had become so anaemic through untreated heavy menstrual bleeding before she consulted me, that she had fainted twice at work!

Encouraging Mrs Weston to talk about herself, she reluctantly admitted to having felt unwell frequently during her periods, and even to taking the occasional aspirin. But she continued to deny that periods can present any sort of a serious problem and, warming to her subject, said that a great deal of unnecessary fuss is made about menstruation nowadays in contrast to years ago; girls and women generally would benefit a great deal by working harder, and putting up with a little understandable discomfort every month. Her final comment was: 'We were too busy in my young day to make a fuss about such things – you'd never think of mentioning it, anyhow! We just got on with our jobs, and if you didn't feel well, you just put up with it!'

To my mind, this way of thinking harks back to the belief that 'women should expect to suffer', and, as many women with this attitude tend to be unsympathetic to young family members and co-workers with troublesome periods, it is a good thing gently to point out to them the widespread medical interest in the subject. With the severe curtailment of today's research grants, very few hospitals or universities would condone the wasting of financial resources and research time on a topic of narrow application and little practical help to large numbers of women. It is in fact the case that a great deal of research has been and is being carried out into menstrual and premenstrual problems, and the medical profession, the media and women generally are becoming better informed on the subject every year.

Individuals of either sex who refuse to recognize menstrual problems as deserving of attention and treatment are of course even less inclined to acknowledge the reality and the significance of the premenstrual syndrome. By the same token, it is regrettably true that a number of doctors, especially the older ones, have entrenched attitudes on the subject, and either refuse treatment for premenstrual symptoms or prescribe tranquillizers for them. One can only speak broadly, for there are many older doctors who do keep abreast of new developments and have years of experience of treating women's cyclical complaints successfully. But medical students are taught much more about such topics nowadays than they were twenty or thirty years ago – and this is why, in many cases, the younger generation of doctors can be relied upon to be more understanding, and therefore in a better position to help premenstrual sufferers, than their older colleagues.

Old habits die hard, and prescribing habits are no exception. As the topic of hormonal treatment has been surrounded for so long by controversy and concern over possible side-effects, it can seem easier and safer to tell the patient to put up with her monthly symptoms, or to prescribe a mild tranquillizer to cope with tension and irritability. This was the experience of Elizabeth Howard, a twenty-year-old art student born in the Channel Islands but resident in this country since the age of fifteen.

She had had little trouble with her periods while she lived at home – but had started to get bad stomach-ache during the first two days of bleeding after she left home and came to stay with her aunt in England. The aunt's GP had treated Elizabeth with a low-dose hormone pill and her trouble had cleared up. But for the past eighteen months she had lived with her boyfriend nearer to college and her new doctor did not believe in prescribing anything at all for the premenstrual symptoms she started to complain of – enlarged, painful breasts, depression and weight gain during the week leading up to her periods. He had at first told her that she should accept that she would feel unwell for a few days every month, because 'all women do'!

Disagreeing with his opinion, Elizabeth returned a month later during a busy surgery and pleaded for help – and was handed a prescription for low-dose Valium tablets. She found these made her sleepy during classes and even more depressed than before. My action was to recommend her to stop taking the tablets forthwith, and write a polite note to her doctor, as I was seeing her privately, informing him that she had discontinued the treatment.

I prescribed diuretic ('water') tablets for five days to give her immediate relief, and advised her to try the new treatment available for the premenstrual syndrome which I shall describe in greater detail later in this book.

One thing is certain: if you suffer from PMS nowadays, you are very unlikely to doubt its existence – provided, of course, that you have heard of it and have been able to identify it, realizing it is a recognized clinical 'syndrome', or complex of interrelated symptoms, in its own right. A distressingly large number of women have never heard of the complaint by name, and so are unaware that their monthly misery, tension and physical symptoms have an underlying physiological cause about which something can now be done. Ruth Elder, for example, whom I saw as an emergency one night when I was on call, knew nothing about the premenstrual syndrome – and although her case was an extreme one it does illustrate the distress, domestic strife and damage that can result when a pronounced case of the illness is unrecognized and left untreated.

Ruth was an Irish girl in her early thirties, and a talented pianist married to a composer and conductor. The couple had two small children, a little girl of five and a baby boy aged two. At first the marriage had been very happy, and Ruth had been full of the joys of life when she had attended surgery for a post-natal examination after the birth of her second child. I hadn't in fact seen her for nearly two years, as she used to bring the children to the Children's Clinic which was held on my day off.

Ruth had been perfectly well until about five months after her son was born, when she started to get depressed and weepy for no apparent reason, and intensely irritable. She tended at times to snap at her music pupils – an essential source of bread and butter while she was continuing to study and audition for work as a concert pianist. Her number of pupils slowly diminished, and a month before I was called to see her, she'd failed an audition she'd set her heart on. The marriage began to show signs of strain, as she often flew off the handle at Anthony, her husband, and at the two children for no reason at all – and Anthony had been retaliating by staying out later and later 'at rehearsals'.

The evening I saw them, her husband informed me that when he had arrived home later than usual, Ruth had gone completely beserk and had attacked him with a carving knife. He had also been very worried earlier in the week at the sight of unexplained bruising on his daughter's back when he had bathed her. When I arrived, Ruth had subsided into floods of tears on the bed, the children were crying in unison and Anthony was beside himself with worry.

I gave Ruth a sleeping tablet, had a chat with her husband, and arranged for him to bring Ruth round to my surgery the next day. There the story unfolded, and was fairly typical of the unsuspected development of the premenstrual syndrome. I explained what the illness consisted of, and told Ruth how to chart her symptoms when they appeared, noting whether her symptoms occurred regularly during the premenstrual phase of her cycle. She was able to tell me there and then that she certainly felt snappier and more moody 'just before the curse was due', and remembered that after failing her audition at which 'she had played appallingly', her period had started the same evening.

Both Ruth and Anthony were back two months later, during which time the children had been staying in the country with Anthony's mother and Ruth had had a rest from teaching and had engaged in minimal performances in public. Showing me her chart, she pointed out that the symptoms tallied in each case with her premenstrual phases. We discussed the premenstrual syndrome in further detail and I recommended a course of self-help treatment for her to follow.

When I saw Ruth three months later she looked very much better. Her husband and the children were happy again – and so was she! She had just won a coveted scolarship which would help financially while she completed her training and she felt on top form again.

As these cases illustrate, several good reasons exist for finding out about the premenstrual syndrome, why it occurs and how it can be treated. There is overwhelming evidence that this illness causes deep unhappiness to thousands of women and consequently to their families as well; also that it causes serious mental and emotional instability in many sufferers. As we strive for, and gradually obtain, equal rights with men on many fronts, naturally we resent more and more bitterly the implication that we are less capable than men, and more likely to go to pieces at regular intervals throughout the course of our reproductive lives. This is not true in the sense that many men think. But it remains true of women who suffer badly from the premenstrual syndrome, all the time the illness remains unrecognized and therefore untreated.

Not all women are affected this way, and ignorance of women's complaints has run full circle. Ironically, just enough is known about female cyclical problems for a great deal of misunderstanding to arise. Many men, employers especially, currently believe that each and every woman is likely to be below par either during her periods or before them or both – and this has an adverse effect upon a woman's chances of obtaining a particular job for which she is well qualified, especially when fellow candidates are male. Increasing numbers of husbands and boyfriends complain, albeit usually tongue-in-cheek, that it is *they* who suffer most from the premenstrual syndrome, since their wives/girlfriends are unliveable-with during the days leading up to their periods. I've even had men come to me asking for tranquillizers for themselves, to be taken during their wives' premenstrual phase every month! What I do under those circumstances, of course, is to ask to see the woman concerned who, though doubtless the cause of marital discord, is invariably suffering far more herself; and I treat her, requesting the man to bear patiently with his wife or lover while we sort her problem out.

It follows from all this, that the more widely knowledge of the premenstrual syndrome is disseminated, the sooner we can hope for an end to prejudice and misunderstanding. If your daughter, mother or best friend, girlfriend or wife, is extraordinarily irritable, perhaps even violent, at times do ask her to consider whether she may be suffering from the premenstrual syndrome. Even bad-tempered, irritable people are easier to live with and love, once you and they understand that there is a reason for the way they feel and behave, particularly now that there is much that can be done to correct the underlying problem.

And, of course, if you suffer from the premenstrual syndrome yourself, it is imperative that you identify the cause of your symptoms so that you can put an end to the problem at the earliest possible opportunity. The good news is that the illness can now be identified for certain, and that the most recently discovered remedy is a natural, drug-free product which you can obtain and administer to yourself with absolute safety.

1

Defining the Premenstrual Syndrome

What exactly is the premenstrual syndrome? Has it only recently come to the notice of the medical profession, or has it been recognized for a long time, even though nothing has been done until recently to estimate the size of the problem and to attempt to alleviate it?

Its definition is: 'a group of physical and mental changes, which begin anything between two and fourteen days before menstruation, and which are relieved almost immediately the period starts'.[1] In many women, mood change is one of the most prominent features, usually to a state of extreme irritability which expresses itself as irrational anger with or without physical violence at one end of the spectrum, and as impatience and snappiness at the other. The subjective feeling accompanying the outward irritability, is one of extreme tension, and women who experience this describe the sensation vividly.

These are some of the comments women have made to me on how the extreme tension affects them: 'I feel as though I am being wound up to snapping point' (thirty-three-year-old mother of two); 'It's as though a metal spring in my solar plexus were being wound up tighter and tighter, until it suddenly snaps' (twenty-year-old medical student); 'I get the sensation of molten liquid heating up inside me, and the more desperately I try to control it, the more it simmers and starts to boil – until suddenly it bursts forth like a stream of molten lava, devastating obstacles in its path' (forty-year-old librarian, with a history of violent outbursts, including physical assault, occurring during the premenstrual phase of her cycle).

It is this symptom of tension which gave the old name of premenstrual tension to the syndrome as a whole; but this in fact is both inaccurate and inadequate because it represents only one characteristic of a plethora of symptoms, and understates the case for women who also suffer from depression, lethargy and numerous physical complaints which we will look at in detail.

Having distinguished between premenstrual tension and the premenstrual syndrome, I should also point out that the latter is a distinct entity from the actual period – as emphasized in the definition above, the premenstrual syndrome is relieved immediately the actual period starts, i.e. bleeding commences. The type of pain associated with the actual period is known as 'spasmodic dysmenorrhoea' – 'spasmodic' due to the manner in which the pains are produced, and 'dysmenorrhoea' simply meaning pain experienced during menstruation. It commences at the same time as the bleeding, and nearly all women have at least some experience of this kind of discomfort. Occurring for the most part in the lower abdomen or the small of the back, spasmodic dysmenorrhoea is a heavy, bloated, dragging feeling, sometimes accompanied by dull or shooting pains in the genital area. One of the best ways to relieve it is to lie still, in bed – either flat on your back on a well-heated underblanket, or curled up on your side with a covered hot-water bottle held close to the affected area. I find this type of discomfort, which can amount to severe pain in some women, responds quite satisfactorily to soluble aspirin, or to aspirin/codeine combinations, and generally resolves itself after the first couple of days of a period.

The cause of spasmodic dysmenorrhoea is directly associated with the changes that the womb (or uterus) undergoes during a period. A period occurs because the lining that the uterus has prepared to ensure the healthy growth of a fertilized egg has not received such an egg to nurture, and requires casting off. This is achieved by the muscular walls of the uterus contracting, and thereby emptying itself of the wasted lining, rather in the way that a tube of toothpaste is emptied by squeezing.

Strong, sustained contraction of muscle fibres is almost always painful, due to the interruption of normal blood flow and the consequent accumulation of chemical substances called metabolites. Spasmodic dysmenorrhoea is sometimes due to the immaturity of the contracting muscles which naturally have difficulty in stretching if they are insufficiently developed. This tends to affect young women and girls most severely during the early months and sometimes years following the onset of their periods, before the uterine muscles have received enough female hormone (oestrogen) to ensure their complete development.

The stretching of the neck of the uterus can also contribute a factor to the total pain experienced during bleeding, as it expands to allow the outward flow of the uterus lining. The reason that such pains are less common after the birth of a baby is that both uterus and muscles are stretched considerably during labour and delivery, and subsequent periods are less demanding on the muscles concerned.

In addition to spasmodic pain, it is also common to feel depressed, headachey and inert during the first two or three days of your period. But actual period pains are quite distinct from the premenstrual syndrome, which has a long list of symptoms both physical and mental, and comes to an abrupt halt just as the period begins, or within an hour or so of its starting. Clearly, if you are unfortunate enough to suffer from both premenstrual symptoms and painful periods, the former may merge into the latter, without so much as a breathing space to allow you to distinguish between them, but fortunately it is uncommon to suffer from both. Another distinguishing feature between the two is that while periods tend to get a lot more tolerable as you get older, the premenstrual syndrome tends to get more severe.

What physical symptoms do sufferers from the premenstrual syndrome complain of? They are numerous and include: swelling of the abdomen, ankles and fingers, and a feeling of being bloated and swollen; weight gain, usually of several pounds but in rare cases of as much as a stone; heavy, engorged, painful breasts; headaches; clumsiness; pain or cramp similar to spasmodic dysmenorrhoea; low urine output; skin disorders such as acne, blotches and whiteheads; and changes in appetite and sleeping requirements.

Mental and emotional symptoms include: tension and irritability; intense depression; lethargy; reduced powers of concentration; illogical emotional reactions; a loss of confidence and feelings of worthlessness and an absence of sex drive. Added to these, the premenstrual syndrome victim may also have to bear with a diminished memory, very poor emotional control, cravings for certain types of food and drink, and diminished work and exercise tolerance, i.e. an abnormal degree of fatigue.

The kind of stomach-ache or low backache, called congestive dysmenorrhoea, which you are likely to experience if you suffer from the premenstrual syndrome is distinct from the spasmodic type already described and is not, strictly speaking, 'dysmenorrhoea' at all as it occurs before – not during – menstruation. It is caused by congestion of the blood vessels in the pelvic and genital regions, and is a dull, persistent pain in contrast to actual period pain. That has the tendency to be cramp-like, i.e. to grow more intense and then diminish alternately, as the muscles of the uterus undergo a sustained contraction, followed by a period of relaxation, followed by yet another pronounced contraction.

In answer to the question: Have we known about the premenstrual syndrome for a long time, or has it only recently come to the notice of the medical profession? – mention of the prominent feature of tension during the premenstrual phase was made in an obscure footnote in medical textbooks as long ago as the seventeenth century. But the syndrome as a whole, and the tension element in particular, did not become headline news until 1981 when two women, both facing charges for serious criminal offences, pleaded suffering from the premenstrual syndrome as an extenuating circumstance, in the defence at their respective trials.

Before we look at these two cases, and at the lighter sentences both women received as a result of this claim, it is helpful to look at the social implications of the premenstrual syndrome generally, since aggression, irrational anger and violent behaviour are prominent features. As many as eighty per cent of women are aware of some degree of premenstrual changes; forty per cent are substantially disturbed by them, and between ten and twenty per

per cent are seriously disabled as a result of the syndrome.[1, 2] This makes it easy to see that a woman suffering from this complaint is not only in need of help herself, but also undergoes mood changes which prove to be a serious stress factor within the context of home life, whether this consists of living with her parents, living with husband or lover, or with a child or children of whom she is either one of two parents or a single parent.

Physical assaults that occur indoors breed misery as well as injury, and often result in counter-violence from a physically stronger man unable to control his temper when attacked. The tendency to assault or batter children, when affected by premenstrual changes, is as tragic for the mother in retrospect as it is for the children at the time of the attack; it is also liable to lead to confrontation with the law or at least the GP and social workers, depending on whether the battering is noticed outside the home and upon the severity of the assault.

The inability to control one's violent rages outside the home, and the consequent assault upon a person outside the family circle, inevitably produces retribution in the form of lawsuits and possible sentencing to imprisonment.

With respect to present divorce rates, there is no doubt that a large number of marriages suffer severely as a result of the woman's premenstrual mood swings and irrational behaviour. So, of course, do they suffer as a result of men's irrational behaviour and tendencies to violence; but in this instance we are looking at the effects of the premenstrual syndrome on marriage, and it is fair to say that a considerable number of the divorces that occur every year are caused in the main by premenstrual rows and physical assault and counter-assault. Women who seek treatment for their premenstrual symptoms are the first to complain that their marriage/family life is being severely disrupted by their illness – and it is frequently this fact more than any other that prompts them to go to their doctors. Here are some cases of women, suffering from the premenstrual syndrome, who have consulted me about their symptoms during the last eighteen months.

Case 1

Anne was a twenty-three-year-old wife of a business executive and had worked as a secretary for her husband's company until they married. It had been a whirlwind romance which had begun after the office Christmas party and culminated in Basil proposing marriage to Ann the following Easter. They had seen a great deal of one another since first going out together, of course, but as Basil was often away for several days at a time on business conferences abroad, the couple had not had the opportunity of spending many days together at a stretch – especially since Ann was living with her parents at the time. They had a June wedding, and all was well for the first few months, after which they started to argue about small matters and later to have real rows. Anne came to see me when she and Basil had been married for just over a year – and they had already considered having a trial separation. Anne felt it was all her fault; she told me that for several years she had felt tense during the week before her period was due, and that her parents and workmates had learned to put up with and humour her. Basil had tried to do so, too; but everything he did got on her nerves. I questioned her about other symptoms, and she admitted to a weight gain of several pounds during the premenstrual week, as well as headaches, blotchy skin and loss of appetite. Emotionally, she felt she was 'quite abnormal' when premenstrual – and admitted that she had thrown a knife at her husband the previous month. We discussed the premenstrual syndrome in general and her symptoms in particular, and Anne agreed that she would try some treatment, as well as taking my advice about sharing her problem with Basil so that he could be helpful during difficult times.

Case 2
Rachel's case was a little more unusual. She had been with the practice for years, and was a likeable forty-two-year-old lesbian who had 'come out' so far as being gay was concerned, and was very proud of the fact that, after years of counselling, depression and loneliness she had at last found the courage to live as she had always longed to live, i.e. with a permanent lover, instead of feeling obliged to make do with a succession of brief clandestine affairs. I had seen her for something trivial about a year before the consultation in question and she had been over the moon, having fallen in love with a girl a few years her junior and set up home with her. This time she looked depressed, tearful and tired – and I

feared that the relationship had not worked out as she had hoped. 'Meg and I are fine', Rachel announced stoutly, 'or we would be, if it were not for my dreadful tempers . . . ' It seemed that the rages, tearful scenes and violent tempers had always been a part of Rachel's premenstrual phase – but had never affected anyone but herself as she worked at home as a freelance journalist and could cry, beat the furniture and feel thoroughly destructive when premenstrual without her irrational anger causing rows. Now it seemed that, as deeply as she loved Meg, on 'bad' days she would shriek at her, throw things and – the night before the consultation – she had struck her lover hard with a plant-pot. Fortunately Meg had suffered no worse than bruises but was very upset indeed, and had cried more or less continuously since. I discussed treatment alternatives with Rachel, which worked for her, and I was pleased to learn that she had no recurrence of the violent premenstrual outbursts – and that she and Meg stayed together.

Case 3

Another patient who was able to find help among the available modern therapies for symptoms of the premenstrual syndrome was Suzi B. She arrived at the surgery in a distraught state one afternoon, and told me that she had been arrested in the high-street supermarket that morning on a charge of shoplifting – to which she admitted. 'I can't think what came over me, Doctor, but I felt compelled to stuff as many extra items into my pockets and handbag as I could fit – without taking much care not to be caught. It was almost as though I had gone out of my mind temporarily.' She had no history of psychiatric disorders, so I questioned her about her menstrual history. She had a few of the physical symptoms, such as weight gain, painful breasts and a blotchy skin, during the three days prior to each period, and a number of emotional troubles including irrational behaviour, as well as severe headaches and sleep disturbances. Suzi was a pleasant girl of nineteen, married for a year, and with a clean record. She did not appeal for leniency on the grounds of diminished responsibility due to the premenstrual syndrome as her husband did not like the idea, but fortunately she was well represented in court and was given a conditional discharge.

Some women become intensely depressed as a result of the premenstrual syndrome, and a case was reported in the weekly newspaper *Doctor* on 4 March, 1982, in which a woman's suicide, by drowning, was blamed on her premenstrual condition. Miss Grace Chalmers had been found dead in the bath by her brother, for whom she had left a note informing him of her intentions. The coroner's officer reported that Miss Chalmers was being treated by her GP for PMT (*sic*) – i.e. premenstrual tension. The pathologist said at the inquest: 'It was a genuine case of PMT. The cause of death was drowning in someone who, as far as I am able to ascertain, was fit and healthy but undoubtedly had premenstrual tension problems'. At the time of the post-mortem, the uterus was in a premenstrual phase.

These few cases – one of which appeared in a weekly newspaper, and the other three whom I saw as patients in surgery, are neither rare nor exceptional. When you consider that eight out of ten of all women of reproductive age experience some degree of the premenstrual syndrome, and between one and two out of the ten are severely incapacitated by this complaint, it is easy to see that the contribution it can make to higher divorce figures, injured children and the rate of criminal offences among women, is considerable.

There is a further way in which severe premenstrual symptoms can contribute towards marital disharmony. Irritability and irrational anger, with or without tendencies to violence, make the week leading up to a woman's period severely trying. If you suffer in this way yourself and, as is the case with many women, come to dread that time of the month when rows appear inevitable, you will not find the situation helped at all by the fact that your libido reaches an all-time low as well. Irritability is bad enough, as are the rows that ensue; but at least under normal circumstances you can kiss and make up – indeed many couples have a good shindy from time to time just to provide an excuse to go to bed and make love with that degree of passion that often follows upon seeing one's partner aroused and flushed, with a deft tongue, a sparkling eye and a devil-may-care, arrogant defiance. There is generally more than an element of play-acting about rows of this type, even if neither partner is consciously aware of his or her need to flare up with anger from time to time in order to stimulate and release sexual passion. But even the bad days that we all go through, on which each partner seems to have got out of bed firmly on the wrong side and remains in the resultant mood all day, can lead to a warm, affectionate kiss and cuddle later in the day or in bed.

However, the rows that arise from a nagging premenstrual woman and escalate as the stressed, angry husband retaliates rarely end in this way, for many women feel an absence of sexual desire at that time, and some literally shudder at the idea of being caressed, petted or embraced by the very man with whom they normally share a caring, joyous and fulfilling sex life.

One such comment made to me by a patient, Pam Y, illustrates the point perfectly. She told me: 'Every month before my period, it's the same story. I get really worked up at the office during the day, but manage not to explode – just. As soon as I get home, I feel better till Eric comes in, then I explode. I'll find anything to yell at him for, from not putting his dirty socks in the linen bin, to carving the joint badly the previous weekend! He's always tired when he gets home – so inevitably he shouts back and we have a dreadful row. Sometimes he even walks out, and eats at the pub, to get away from me. But we can't make it up in bed, although he attempts to, because my whole attitude at that time, is 'Noli me tangere', and there is nothing I can do about it.'

Once the cause of periodic outbursts, weepiness and nagging can be identified as psychological changes during the premenstrual phase of a woman's cycle, she generally feels better – particularly when she ceases to feel 'freakish' and 'isolated' – and comes to believe that her symptoms may perhaps have a remedy. Her husband, lover and/or family also tend to feel relieved that a clinical explanation exists for what they see as inexplicable and irrational behaviour in a normally well-balanced partner or mother, and on the whole offer understanding and practical help, once they are reassured that outside help is available. This is one of the reasons why you should make every effort to discover whether your recurrent 'blues', irritability or family rows are due to premenstrual syndrome symptoms; if you are concerned about someone else, you should encourage them to find this out for themselves. Even before you take steps to remedy the underlying cause, there is immense therapeutic value in knowing that help is at hand. Treating the premenstrual syndrome effectively and on a widespread basis also has the bonus of combating the notion that women are unreliable and prone to irrational behaviour, and thereby alleviating some of the difficulties some women experience when competing with men for high-powered, executive jobs. Irrational behaviour, a proneness to accidents and poor powers of concentration are experienced by large numbers of women during their premenstrual phases. But this does not make women *per se* less competent than men; it simply makes diagnosis and treatment of the causative condition imperative.

Now let's look at the two cases mentioned above, in which symptoms of the premenstrual syndrome were accepted as grounds for diminished responsibility in two women charged with serious criminal offences. One of these, Mrs Christine English, a thirty-seven-year-old divorced mother of two, killed her lover after an argument by running him over with her car. As he was walking away from her just before the accident, he mocked her by giving her a V-sign. When interviewed by the police afterwards, Mrs English stated that she was already mad at him, and then when this happened she 'just snapped' and jammed her foot on the accelerator, intending to bump into him and hurt him and shut him up – not to kill him.

She was suffering from premenstrual symptoms at the time and claimed this fact as grounds of diminished responsibility. The court accepted her claim and she was given a conditional discharge for twelve months and banned from driving for the same period. It was accepted that Mrs English committed this serious crime 'under wholly exceptional circumstances'.

The second case involved a twenty-nine-year-old barmaid called Sandie Smith. She was put on probation for three years after threatening to kill a policeman with a knife, while already on probation for stabbing a nineteen-year-old girl to death the previous year. The judge told the court that Sandie was not responsible for her actions, 'because her illness had affected her brain'. Said to become like a 'raging animal' when affected by the premenstrual syndrome, Sandie told reporters as she left the Old Bailey: 'This is the end of a nightmare for me. I am glad it is all over. *I never knew why I turned violent. I'm hoping to start a new life now that I'm free.*'

The italics in the above quotation are mine, because what

Sandie Smith said is very significant. There is no doubt that she was referring to freedom from criminal charges and imprisonment. But she had been freed in another, even more important, sense; she had learned that her bodily changes at the time of the premenstrual phase of her cycle lessened her normal self-control to the point at which 'she was not responsible for her actions'. And instead of being at the mercy of her own irrational and destructive outbursts, she was at liberty to receive treatment, thereby ceasing to be the unwilling victim, while at the same time the perpetrator, of violent tendencies.

As often happens when a criminal case or series of cases make headline news and the ensuing sentence reflects an unexpected liberality on behalf of the judge, controversy raged for some time over the sentences these two women received, on account of the degree of leniency shown. This was welcomed by a large number of people on behalf of all the women who do suffer from violent tendencies during the premenstrual phase, and this view was backed up by the findings of one study carried out on inmates of Holloway Women's Prison. It was revealed that nearly fifty per cent of the prisoners had committed their crimes within four days of menstruation.

Other people were less pleased by the enlightened approach of the judges, for they were concerned that these cases might set dangerous precedents. The problem was that although, in the past, courts had agreed to take into account the defendant's state of health when the crime was committed, it had always been by way of mitigation, i.e. it was a factor capable of affecting leniency of the sentence being passed. The proceedings of these two cases, however, appeared to propose that the premenstrual syndrome should be a special defence absolving women suffering from it from any liability whatever for their criminal activities. The only precedent for such a blanket defence is insanity; but in order to protect society from those on whose behalf this defence is claimed, the law imposes a number of privations on the insane persons concerned, including, often, the deprivation of freedom. So it was argued by the cynically minded that, if women 'wanted' to be able to lapse into bouts of PMT (sic) inspired criminal instability once a month with impunity, they should not be surprised if the privilege for such a defence cost them some of their other rights.

Sandie Smith appealed against her conviction in April of the following year. The Court of Appeal heard how the premenstrual syndrome had turned her into an uncontrollable 'Jeckyll and Hyde', whose behaviour was 'incredibly abnormal'. It was further claimed, on Sandie's behalf, that she had committed the crimes 'without the willpower to stop her actions' and 'without knowing what she was doing'. It was suggested that the premenstrual syndrome should, as a matter of policy, be accepted as a valid defence in a criminal court. The Court of Appeal, however, and in particular Lord Justice Griffiths, was not prepared to 'take a leap in the dark, and make a special defence of someone suffering from the premenstrual syndrome'. He pointed out that, although a court could feel sympathy for a woman unable to control her violent impulses which resulted from the premenstrual syndrome, the purpose of criminal law was to protect society – and protecting society was of greater priority than preventing women from being unfairly branded as criminals. A woman who killed, and was then acquitted on the grounds of premenstrual symptoms, would continue to be 'a danger to all around her'.

The premenstrual syndrome remains, then, for the time being, a mitigating factor and is not included with insanity as a blanket defence.[3]

The best thing to result from this decision is that it underlines the crucial point that severe premenstrual syndrome changes unleash the bonds of control, so that innate tendencies to violent behaviour demonstrate themselves in actions which would virtually never be performed under other circumstances, regardless of provocation.

Claire Rayner states in *Woman's Own*:

> . . . you have no need to fear that you will become a raving maniac overnight . . . women who suffer from [the premenstrual syndrome] are likely to react as they always do, *but in an exaggerated way*. The woman who becomes tearful under stress will cry even more; the one who reacts with fury, will lose her temper more quickly, and so on.

By and large this is true. But at the extreme end of the spectrum there are women whose behaviour and feelings run so far out of control and are so in contrast to their normal actions and standards during their premenstrual phase that their lives are very severely disrupted. As one patient put it to me: 'I feel a stranger to my husband and family when I am waiting for my period to start – worse than that, I feel unsure of myself, I can't trust myself not to fight and row, whereas normally I am definitely a peacemaker.'

The premenstrual syndrome, by all accounts, is uncomfortable, miserable and isolating – and brings out the worst side in all of us. The next thing to do is to take a detailed look at the physical and mental symptoms, and work out a checklist by which you can ascertain whether or not you are suffering from it.

[1] Dalton, K. *The Premenstrual Syndrome* (Heinemann, 1964).
[2] Reid, R. L. and Yen, S. C.C. 'Premenstrual Syndrome', *American Journal of Obstetrics and Gynaecology* 139, (1981) pp.85-104.
[3] 'The Monthly Syndrome', *Newsweek* (4 May 1981), pp.74-75.

2

The Physical Symptoms

If you are a premenstrual syndrome sufferer, you may well find it difficult to decide whether it is the physical or the psychological symptoms which trouble you the most. The majority of women would probably claim that they find the psychological manifestations, such as extreme tension and uncontrollable irritability, the most intolerable, since these affect many aspects of their lives – in particular, their ability to cope with their jobs and their relationships with their families.

As I mentioned earlier, it is more often psychological changes which finally tip the scales in favour of visiting the doctor, especially when the woman realizes that her moods are sparking off a series of domestic rows. But with respect to the syndrome's physical symptoms, one of the commonest to result in medical consultations is the bloatedness and weight gain which are due to fluid retention during the premenstrual phase.

Weight gain
Most women's weight increases by a couple of pounds for a day or so prior to their periods. In fact, this is so common that most advice on the subject of slimming warns dieters to weigh themselves on a

weekly rather than on a daily basis, because most people's weight fluctuates for a variety of physiological reasons from one day to another; and points out that women's weight can rise, due to the retention of fluid, by several pounds in the days leading up to menstruation. If you suffer badly from premenstrual changes, your weight may increase by as much as half a stone – and I have known at least three women to experience weight gain in the region of twelve to fourteen pounds premenstrually.

Unless you are very slim, any weight gain is annoying, particularly when you have not over-indulged in anything very fattening and so have done nothing to deserve it. If you are one of the millions of women who engage in a constant weight battle and never seem to reach target weight, the premenstrual syndrome may very well be the cause. A common cycle of events is as follows: as a period comes to an end and you start to feel better, your weight also returns – or has already returned, during the first day or so of bleeding – to 'normal', by which I mean that you have little or no excess weight due to fluid retention. Your strong food cravings, which are also a common feature of premenstrual trouble and which I shall deal with in the next chapter, have also disappeared; and you are not feeling tense and unhappy. You stick to your chosen diet satisfactorily for the following two weeks or so, and lose several pounds. Then, let's say, your premenstrual syndrome symptoms start each month about a week before your period is due to begin. You weigh yourself, and your weight is static or, worse still, has increased. Nearly always devastating to the determination of all but the most dedicated slimmer. At the same time, your food cravings get underway, and you positively yearn for all the things you usually deny yourself, such as cream-filled chocolate bars, condensed milk or cream doughnuts. You snap at someone and the ensuing row, coupled with your premenstrual headache, makes you need immediate consolation – so you turn to the cake tin or store cupboard for comfort. Once you have done so, you may well eat in an abandoned way right up to the day your period starts. Then, feeling better, losing some of your excess weight as the fluid leaves your body, and no longer needing excess food, you start all over again on the same predictable course.

If this description fits your eating habits – don't despair. You can avoid the pitfalls of overeating and lose your excess weight – and keep it off. We will go into how this is done later in the book.

Besides the undesirable weight gain and diet interference which result from your body retaining extra fluid, other consequences are passing less urine than usual, and the uncomfortable 'bloated' feeling which makes your clothes feel tight and your stomach enormous. Some women have come to me complaining of feeling and, they feared, looking, several months pregnant when their premenstrual syndromes were in full swing. Few actually look anything like as obviously swollen up as they suppose, but it is certainly true that ordinary skirt and trouser bands feel several sizes too small and less shapely garments have to be resorted to. Your ankles and feet are likely to become puffy, particularly by the end of the day if you are on your feet a lot; and another uncomfortable effect is the tightness of watch-straps, bracelets and rings. Some women have to abandon regularly worn jewellery when premenstrual; others, who refuse to remove treasured rings, often have a very uncomfortable time.

When the retained fluid occupies tissues which cannot expand readily, however, severe pain rather than enlargement may result. If it collects in the tissues of the eyeballs, the eyes can hurt a great deal, and have an increased tendency to become infected. The eye pain can induce headaches, which we will look at in more detail later in this chapter.

Painful breasts
Enlarged painful breasts are another frequent symptom of the premenstrual syndrome, and the degree of discomfort can range from increased sensitivity to acute tenderness. Generally, the breasts are just as affected by the retention of fluid as the rest of the body, but they are a favourite place for it to collect, and since they are sensitive at the best of times and bras tend to be close-fitting garments, an increase in the size of the breasts is felt by the bra becoming considerably tighter. Their increased awareness of touch can make you most anxious to avoid picking anything up, hugging anyone, or doing anything which will involve their being pressed.

If your breasts are affected in this way, you may be tempted to abandon your bra and 'go easy' in a large, sloppy sweater; but this can often be as bad, in a different way, since the increased heaviness of the breast tissue will make you very aware of their movement underneath your clothes, and their being bumped around can be even worse than a too-tight bra, which at least supports them.

There are two reasons for the acute breast tenderness associated with the premenstrual syndrome. The first is obvious – the pressure caused by the excess fluid present in the tissues. The second is the fact that the blood supply to them increases at this time, and the greater blood flow through the skin and underlying tissues increases their sensitivity considerably.

Some women who are not aware of the extent to which the premenstrual phase can affect their breasts can become seriously worried by the acute discomfort they experience every month. It is an area of the body about which women worry anyway, because of the association with breast lumps and cancer – and I have seen one or two young girls extremely frightened by the fact that their breasts were painful.

June Summers was a seventeen-year-old who came to the surgery accompanied by a schoolfriend, who explained what was the matter – June seemed too scared to speak. As soon as I learned that the breast pain recurred every month, and disappeared as soon as her period started, I was able to reassure her – and my examination of her breasts confirmed that there was nothing for her to worry about. She had plucked up courage to come, as she was preparing for GCE A-levels and the worry had been preventing her from studying.

This is yet another indication of the need for more information on the premenstrual syndrome being made available. Even knowing how to examine your own breasts for lumps does not always put the mind at rest on the subject, as premenstrual breast swelling can accentuate the natural granular feel some normal breast tissue has, and can be worrying to the woman concerned. In a similar way, the excess fluid can increase the size of completely benign (i.e. harmless) breast lumps, which have already been diagnosed as innocent, and women return to the surgery time and again, afraid that their 'lump' has suddenly turned into cancer, because it is larger and painful.

On this score, it is worth remembering that the breast pain and swelling that occur regularly and only during the week before your period starts, and disappear when your period arrives, can safely be put down to the premenstrual syndrome. It is also worth remembering that if a breast lump hurts, and you can wiggle it around in your breast, it is extremely likely to be a benign lump. Check with your doctor anyway, to make certain. But the lump to worry about — or rather, not to worry about, but to consult your doctor about without a moment's loss – is the hard, irregular, painless one.

Headaches

Headaches are another common feature of the premenstrual syndrome, and some women dread that phase of their cycle on this account. There are many different types of headache, and very many reasons why they occur, so I always try to remember to check the regularity with which this symptom is experienced and, in the case of a woman of reproductive age, whether they are related to her premenstrual phase.

Premenstrual headaches are generally of two different varieties, and this fact makes it easier to identify and to treat them. The first affects the face as much as, if not more than, it does the head. It is a constant, often severe pain affecting the top of the head and the forehead, the cheekbones, the eyes and occasionally the upper teeth. This type is in fact another symptom of fluid retention and is largely due to the sinuses being blocked by swollen cells. The passage of air through the nasal channels also becomes blocked, so in addition to headaches like this you may well get a stuffy nose and difficulty in breathing.

The second kind of typical premenstrual headache is the tension variety. As we have seen, tension is one of the cardinal features of the illness, and a typical tension headache consists of a throbbing pain in the forehead and the sensation of a metal band growing tighter and tighter around the head. Everyday stresses frequently bring on 'stress headaches', and the premenstrual syndrome accentuates the effects that stress has on those who suffer from it.

Migraine attacks

Migraine attacks can occur as part of the premenstrual illness. Established migraine sufferers have an increased chance of getting an attack during this time; other people get migraine attacks only during this time, and never at any other.

As is the case with tension headaches, migraine attacks and the pain they produce are caused by the contraction of the blood vessels supplying the brain, followed by a relaxation phase. We will take a closer look at just what causes this common and very unpleasant aspect of the premenstrual phase when we examine the causes of the premenstrual syndrome as a whole. The initial pain is usually a throbbing sensation occurring on one side of the head only, and slowly increasing until the entire head is involved. The throbbing generally gives way to a persistent ache, which can vary in intensity from the merely unpleasant to the frankly agonizing. Premenstrual migraine attacks are preceded and accompanied by the same types of symptoms as 'ordinary' migraine attacks, i.e. an aura can occur before the attack, when the vision is affected and the patient experiences partial blindness and / or flashing, coloured lights. Nausea and vomiting affect many women, and so does photophobia (increased visual sensitivity to light).

Rosalind Morison, a twenty-year-old nurse working for the practice, finds that she can continue with her work and get through a migrainous premenstrual day, providing she can 'catch' an attack early enough by means of taking pain-killers at the first possible sign that an attack is about to start. If she ignores the early warning – in her case, flashing purple and yellow lights which she sees out of the corners of her eyes – and the actual headache gets a hold, she has to lie down in a dark room for the rest of the day, and gets profuse vomiting as well.

A proneness to accidents

Clumsiness and an increased proneness to accidents is a proven factor of the premenstrual syndrome. This refers not only to accidents outside the home, when you are using machinery or driving a car, but also an increased tendency to drop things, cut yourself, bang into doors or hard objects (exceptionally irritating!) and even to trip and fall, or overbalance while on steps and ladders.

In some factories this tendency is recognized, and women are given different jobs away from dangerous machinery during their premenstrual weeks. Many nasty accidents have been avoided by this measure. When the Medical Committee on Accident Prevention carried out a study on women involved in car accidents, they discovered that instead of the twenty-five per cent which you would expect to occur in any one of the four weeks of the monthly cycle, the premenstrual week accounted for as many as forty-eight per cent. Findings of another study by the same committee revealed that accidents are far commoner during the premenstrual phase than at any other time, as evidenced by the increase in hospital admissions and visits to the doctor's surgery during that time.

Since I am particularly interested in women's complaints and especially in the premenstrual syndrome, I make a point of asking women of reproductive age who come to my surgery with small burns, scalds, knife cuts, grazes and lacerations etc., whereabouts they are in their monthly cycles. Over a three-year period, I have discovered that, of 223 such women, ninety-three of them were premenstrual, that is, just over forty-two per cent.

Precise explanations have not been forwarded for increased clumsiness and accident proneness during the premenstrual phase, but most authorities agree that relevant factors are an increase in muscular tension which occurs as a result of the inner tensions, coupled with poor concentration and lethargy. If you feel inert and unwilling to exert yourself, you tend to be careless, and hurry through jobs to get them over and done with, or from place to place, to put the journey behind you as soon as possible.

Aches and pains

We have looked at the congestive dysmenorrhoea problem and how it arises; this accounts for the low backache and the persistent, low, dragging abdominal pain which may affect you during the days leading up to your period.

The other aches and pains are those involving muscles and joints, and they have two main causes. One of these is the increased pressure within the tissues as retained fluid starts to collect there, pressing on nerve endings and thereby causing pain. The other is the increased state of tension of the muscle fibres themselves which may be due to the way in which the actual muscle cells are affected by the premenstrual changes, or may simply relate to a woman's personal increase in inner tension.

If you are feeling cross, headachey and stressed almost to breaking point, then it is very hard to relax and unconsciously all your muscles are held in a state of increased tension. Your muscular 'tone' reflects your general state of well-being, and you will invariably find that when you feel happy and carefree you also suffer fewer aches and pains. This is because messages from your brain are no longer conveying a state of danger alert to your muscles, and they do not therefore hold themselves in a state of tension, ready for 'flight or fight'. They resume their normal tone and their blood supply is adequate, allowing nourishment to reach the muscle fibres and the toxic substances (metabolites) to be carried away. When a muscle is held in a state of tension for prolonged periods, it 'clamps down' on its own blood supply and the metabolites collect within the substance of the muscle. Insufficient oxygen is brought to the muscle by the lowered blood supply and it is the presence of the resultant metabolites which causes the pain.

Skin disorders

Skin disorders are one of the more minor effects of the premenstrual syndrome in most women who suffer from it. They find that they have an increased tendency to develop acne during the premenstrual week, and generally their skin is blotchy, shows a number of blemishes and whiteheads and looks less than its best. They may also notice patches of unexplained bruising.

An increased tendency to allergies has been shown to be associated with the illness, and it is thought that this may account in part for the poor condition of the skin at this time.

The spots and blemishes usually clear up quickly once the period has started. Probably the worst aspect of the skin disorder is the effect it has on the woman's morale at this time. It is bad enough to feel irritable, depressed, inert, clumsy and bloated; it can be the last straw (or seem like it) to look in the mirror, where we often turn for reassurance, and have our suspicions confirmed that we really are looking at our worst!

Abnormal cravings

I have discussed the abnormal food cravings one can get at this time. Besides the need to derive some comfort from a reliable source because you are feeling low, a physiological reason seems to play a part in some women's cravings for sweet, starchy food items before their periods start. The changes that occur in the body during this time can cause a fall in the blood sugar level. When this occurs, your nervous system registers the fact and the message your brain receives, and which you interpret, is for the need for an increase in the sugar supply – fast. You crave sweet things and many women give in to this certainly very strong urge.

The other abnormally strong urge is for sleep. If you are at work all day or have young children to look after, then you doubtless have to fight the strong desire to nod off and resort to numerous cups of coffee or perhaps cigarettes to keep you awake. If you are at home all day alone you may very well go to sleep for long periods – only to wake up unrefreshed and probably with a headache.

Neither stimulants nor abnormally long sleeping hours is the answer to this problem. It can only be solved by treating the premenstrual syndrome as a whole.

3

The Psychological Symptoms

Now let's take a closer look at the psychological symptoms of the premenstrual syndrome. It is likely, but not inevitable, that you will experience psychological changes if you do suffer from this illness; a few women notice only the physical discomforts which we looked at in the previous chapter. Others, however, experience only the emotional turmoil of premenstrual change, and it is these women who may find it harder to identify the premenstrual syndrome as the cause of their trouble.

If you are overweight, spotty and have painful breasts and migraine attacks, on a regularly recurrent basis, you are likely to want to find out whether there is a physical cause. If, however, you suffer from none of these complaints but experience instead recurrent rages, depression, food cravings and bouts of poor concentration, then you are less likely to look for a physical explanation for your complaints.

The psychological changes are, therefore, considerably more subtle than the physical ones, and can lead to a great deal of misery, self-doubt and misjudgement by others – unless and until it is established that it is not your personality which is at fault, but a series of chemical changes in your body over which you have no control.

One fact that emerges from all this should be emphasized, since it is a very important one. Your personal version of the premenstrual syndrome is unlikely to be identical to that of your best friend or, for that matter, to those of the girls at work or to the premenstrual condition of your next-door neighbour. Every woman who suffers from the premenstrual syndrome has her own particular premenstrual syndrome profile. So it is essential that you do not prejudge the issue and decide that you could not possibly be suffering from this illness because your symptoms do not tally with those of someone else you know who is already a confirmed sufferer.

Similar to the physical symptoms, the psychological changes which can be caused by premenstrual illness have their own spectra of severity, at any point on which your own particular experience of it may lie. Tension may be mild or severe; concentration may be slightly affected or severely impaired; and irritability, as we saw in Chapter 2, ranges from shortness of temper to homicidal rage.

You can help yourself to obtain a clear picture of how, exactly, you are affected, by referring to the checklist of symptoms and filling in the charts detailed later in this book, with your own personal data. Once you are quite certain that you are indeed suffering from the premenstrual syndrome – because your symptoms always start while you are waiting for your period to begin, and disappear soon after bleeding commences – then you are in a position to do something about them.

Tension

There is always a thin dividing line between the workings of our minds and the workings of our bodies, and tension gives rise to a number of physical symptoms as well as generating a good deal of mental distress. As I mentioned when discussing aches and pains in the last chapter, mental tension generates a hyper-tense condition in your muscles, and leads to stiffness, clumsiness and aching limbs and joints. Increased muscular tension is one of the aspects of the 'flight or fight' reflex mechanism, and is associated with an increased outpouring of adrenalin by your adrenal glands.

Increased adrenalin levels in the blood are also responsible for a pounding heartbeat, an uncomfortably dry mouth and shallow, rapid breathing. Mentally you feel completely 'wound up' and, as some of the case histories quoted earlier in this book indicate, it takes very little stress to cause you to lose control.

Here is another case in which the patient's chief problem was one of premenstrual tension. Her words further clarify the bad experience that this can prove. Phyllis, a thirty-two-year-old shop assistant, came to see me to ask for tranquillizers. She had never been on them before, but she was finding that the recurrent tension which she experienced in the premenstrual phase of her cycle, was making life very difficult for her at work.

Working in a shop can be incredibly tiring, as you will know if you have ever tried it, and Phyllis was used to painful feet and aching swollen ankles at the end of the day, which is why she had not consulted me before. She was also used to headaches from the fluorescent lighting; and to nasal stuffiness, which she attributed to the central heating. None of these symptoms of fluid retention had given her a clue to the fact that she was suffering from the premenstrual syndrome.

Phyllis found that she was 'ratty' sometimes with her workmates, but in general remained on good terms with them. She had recently been worried, however, by the fact that she was becoming irritable with the customers, and on the day that she came to see me (a dark, cold day during the January sales), she had had to leave work early on account of tension symptoms.

'All those customers, shoving and pushing one another,' she said. 'We all know what the sales are like, and expect crowds of people – in fact, I even used to enjoy it! But today I felt that they were pressing in on me and that any moment I was going to scream and lash out at them. I told the manageress that I had a bad headache and went home. But it was the same in the rush before Christmas, and I'm finding that I can't cope.'

Careful questioning about physical and psychological health revealed the fact that Phyllis was getting her symptoms during her premenstrual weeks only, and I was able to suggest a course of action to her which helped her a great deal.

Irritability
This, as we have seen, is the outward expression of inner tension, and productive of much domestic strife and personal misery. It

also sometimes results in physical violence, and it was this that
brought Maureen, a likeable thirty-year-old mother of four, to see
me as an emergency appointment one morning. Things had got so
bad at home that she had walked out, leaving everything in the
hands of a neighbour, and had come straight along to the surgery
to see me, even forgetting to remove her apron.

Her first words to me were that she would like me to have her
children taken into care. We all know Maureen and her children at
the surgery, and she is normally an excellent and caring parent; so
I asked the receptionist to make her a cup of tea and I gave her a
single Valium tablet to help calm her down. She was then better
able to tell me her troubles.

'Every so often I get very snappy with the kids,' she admitted,
'and this morning was the last straw. Kevin was sick and couldn't
go to nursery school, the baby as you know has got measles, and
Roy rang up just after he got to work to say that his hours have
been cut again, which means less money of course, just after we'd
signed the HP agreement for the new carpets.

'Just as I put the receiver down, Lorraine dropped one of my
best vases and broke it, and knocked the goldfish bowl over at the
same time. All the kids started to scream and the cat got one of the
goldfish; and what with the screaming, the flapping fish and water
everywhere, I went mad.

'I kicked the cat, really hard, only managed to save two of the
goldfish, and shook Lorraine so roughly I'm sure her teeth rattled.
At this moment I feel that I could take a gun to the whole lot of
them, so it's only right that they should be removed before I can
do them any serious harm.'

I calmed her down, and pointed out gently that she had not
done any of the children any real harm. I reminded her that she
had coped with worse family crises before. She even managed to
see the funny side of the domestic scene that had driven her mad –
especially when I was able to tell her that I was certain that she was
suffering from the premenstrual syndrome and that there was a
great deal that could be done to alleviate the symptoms of tension
and irritability.

It turned out that she was expecting her next period to start that
very day; and she remembered that she had had a row with her
husband and had got very angry with the children at exactly the

same point in her cycle the previous month. Maureen had never heard of the premenstrual syndrome, and was deeply relieved to hear that her outbursts of anger and moodiness could be attributed to an illness for which treatment existed.

Depression
Depression is another common feature of the premenstrual syndrome. Before the latter was recognized as a clinical entity, a number of depressed women were sent to psychiatrists and received anti-depressant drugs and tranquillizers for depressive illness which was occurring rather as a symptom of an underlying disorder than as true depressive disease *per se*.

Now, depression – varying in intensity from monthly 'blues' to severe and suicidal desperate misery – is recognized as a cardinal feature of the illness. One of the characteristics of premenstrual depression is the rapidity with which it can strike a normally equable and happy woman as the internal changes commensurate with the syndrome start to come into play. In fact, mood swings, i.e. changes from normal cheerfulness to severe misery, tearfulness and irritability, are characteristic of this illness.

Just 'feeling down' can be bad enough. A low mood, coupled with feeling uncomfortable and unattractive, makes some women overeat and others turn to rather too many drinks in order to find consolation. Severe depression is a devastating experience, and when experiencing it at its worst, it is not uncommon to revert to what amounts to a foetal state in which all hope, desire and appreciation of life are lost; and the overwhelming craving is for perpetual silence, darkness and oblivion.

There is in fact an unconscious irony in the statements of many depressed people, namely, that the only reason that they do not commit suicide is that they have not sufficient motivation or energy to do so. Depression of this severity is an emergency and requires accurate diagnosis and immediate treatment.

When the depression lacks an apparent underlying cause, such a degree of illness is usually treated on an 'in-patient' basis, by means of an intensive course of anti-depressant drugs and/or electro-convulsive therapy (electric shock treatment). Counselling and psychotherapy are introduced at a later stage, when the person is sufficiently receptive to be able to benefit from them.

When severe depression is part of the premenstrual syndrome, and occurs regularly in the premenstrual phase, the woman's mood returning to normal as, or just after, her period starts, then it is the premenstrual illness itself and not the symptomatic depression which requires therapy. Tranquillizers and sedatives dampen you down and are not indicated in depression. In fact, Valium has the causation of depression as a recognized side-effect in some people! – and any drug that worsens the depressive state is clearly the last thing that should be given.

When a course of anti-depressant drugs is given, it is generally seven to ten days before benefit is felt. This is because a certain concentration of the drug has to be present in the blood, for a minimum period of time, before its effects are felt. Since the depression associated with premenstrual illness is necessarily short-lived, lasting between two and fourteen days every month, there is no point in prescribing an antidepressant drug on an unsatisfactory 'on-off' basis.

If you get severely depressed in the way I have described, do make every effort when you are *not* depressed to discover whether the premenstrual syndrome is responsible. You are then in a position to do something about your problem.

Aspects of depression which commonly affect premenstrual syndrome sufferers, include feelings of deep unworthiness, an absence of sex drive and severely depleted self-confidence. We have looked at the loss of libido which may occur and noted how it may contribute to marital discord; there is not a great deal to say about the other symptoms, except that they are very unpleasant and distressing, and should constitute a strong incentive to have your premenstrual illness sorted out at the earliest possible opportunity.

Lethargy

Lethargy is frequently found in women suffering from the premenstrual syndrome, mainly those who tend to get very depressed during this time. This is probably because lethargy is a very common feature in ordinary depressive illness, so it is hard to be sure whether the lethargy occurring in the premenstrual syndrome is part of the depression experienced, or a separate feature.

Certainly feelings of lethargy and inertia go hand in hand with prolonged fatigue, and you may well feel extremely tired, after surprisingly little exertion, during your premenstrual days.

Avril Honeyman, a twenty-five-year-old copywriter, told me: 'I work in a bright, creative office where everybody is very lively and on the ball. Usually, I am that way, too, and keep well up to date with my work schedules.

'During the ten days or so before my period starts each month, however, I get slower and slower, and feel lethargic and tired, no matter how many early nights I manage. I find that I'm working more and more slowly – and the effort to turn out even a few lines of second-rate copy, every hour, is enormous. I try to buck myself up by drinking lots of coffee and smoking, and keeping the window near my desk wide open. But nothing seems to help.

'A number of people in our company are going to be made redundant at the end of next month. I'm really afraid that I will be one of them, if I can't find an answer to my problem.'

Reduced powers of concentration
Jane Winter, a twenty-four-year-old medical student, came to see me three months before she was due to sit her Final examinations. This is her story.

'I am getting desperate because I think I am probably suffering from the premenstrual syndrome but haven't found a way to overcome it. I can cope with the physical symptoms and have been given diuretic tablets for fluid retention. These don't help for long, and my chief problem is reduced powers of concentration.

'Finals are thirteen weeks away, and we are all burning midnight oil at the moment – or trying to. The trouble is that as soon as I sit down at my desk in the evening when I am premenstrual, I start studying and almost at once I am day-dreaming. I wake up half an hour later to find that I have done nothing. It happens time and again, and affects me for about ten days at a time. This means that between now and the Finals, I will have about thirty days in which my mental powers will be very much reduced. Can you help?

'I also find that it is far harder than usual to remember facts, if I do succeed in concentrating for a few minutes on the page of a textbook.'

Poor concentration and memory are familiar aspects of the premenstrual syndrome, and they can only be remedied by treating the underlying complaint.

4

Why Does It Happen?

Now that we have been into the signs and symptoms of the premenstrual syndrome in some depth, it is clearly very exciting news that a fresh nutritional approach is producing excellent results in women suffering from this complaint. In order to understand what the new therapy involves, however, and how it works, it is necessary to see how the syndrome comes about in the first place.

Why do some women suffer from the premenstrual syndrome – or, for that matter from the traditional 'curse' of difficult periods – while others have no bother at all? The reason, of course, is individual variation. Just as every one of us has some slight physical defect on the exteriors of our bodies – for instance, one leg half-an-inch shorter than the other, moles on our faces, or a missing toe or finger – so also can internal organs, and the internal systems composed not of organs but of chemical substances, be less than perfect.

Too much or too little of a given hormone, digestive juice or blood constituent, may be produced by a group of cells or a gland, and this can throw an entire chemical system off balance.

The chemical substances involved in menstrual and premenstrual function are, of course, the hormones. But you may have noticed that, so far, I have avoided the use of the word in almost every instance, whereas you might have expected me to use it a great deal when discussing the premenstrual syndrome. This was because I did not want to give the impression that premenstrual symptoms are exclusively hormonally generated, before I was in a position to qualify the statement. This may come as a surprise, as the premenstrual syndrome has always been considered a hormonal problem by all those people who attached any real credence to it in the first place. And it is certainly true that hormone levels play a major part in the whole picture.

But it is now believed that the basic cause of the trouble is a deficiency, within the body of the affected women, of substances called essential fatty acids (EFAs), and that the hormonal imbalance is an apparent, not a real, one, due to this particular deficiency.

Before we go into this topic, we should look at the hormones themselves, and remind ourselves how they are involved in the monthly cycle.

Normal monthly cycle
The focal point of your monthly menstrual cycle is ovulation, which is the shedding of a mature egg ready for fertilization. This is controlled by hormones produced by the pituitary gland in the brain – namely follicle stimulating hormone (FSH) and luteinizing hormone (LH).

The pituitary gland is, in turn, under the control of the hypothalamus, an area in the brain about the size of a greengage, where the control centre of the menstrual cycle is located. The pituitary gland sits just under the hypothalamus and communicates with it through strands of nerve tissue.

The egg is contained in a small pocket in the ovary, called the ovarian follicle, and this ripens under the influence of FSH. As it does so, it secretes the hormone oestrogen, which causes the lining of the womb, or uterus, to thicken up from its thin, post-menstrual condition.

When the oestrogen has reached a certain level in the blood, the little pocket, or follicle, ruptures, the egg is shed into the Fallopian tube, the pituitary gland stops producing FSH and produces LH instead.

The little follicle area on the ovary becomes known as the corpus luteum after the egg has been discharged from it, and it now produces mainly progesterone and only a little oestrogen. This latter aids the thickening process of preparing the lining of the uterus to receive and care for a fertilized egg.

If the egg passes along the Fallopian tubes and into the uterus without being fertilized by a sperm, then the corpus luteum becomes smaller and dies away and the progesterone level in the blood falls. This starts about day twenty-two of the cycle, and is followed by the lining being shed together with the unfertilized egg, starting around day twenty-eight. This is your period.

One widespread and popular theory about the cause of the premenstrual syndrome, is that it is due to a deficiency of progesterone. This belief found a great deal of support for years and progesterone therapy became one of the most usual methods of treating the complaint. Careful scrutiny of the evidence, however, suggests that there is little real foundation for this hypothesis since progesterone therapy appears to be ineffective in most women.[1] Another reason for doubt is that there is not consistent lowering of the progesterone levels in women suffering from premenstrual symptoms. If low levels of this hormone were found in all, or nearly all, of the women who suffer from this illness, then it would be reasonable to suppose this particular hormonal deficiency to be a major causative factor. It would probably also be the case, were this true, that giving progesterone to women suffering from the premenstrual syndrome, would be much more effective than it in fact is.

It is certainly true that progesterone levels are low in some women who suffer from premenstrual illness, and a number of them do benefit from taking a progesterone supplement. But many women with severe premenstrual disorders are found to have normal progesterone levels, and this is why we cannot say with accuracy that it is primarily a lack of this hormone which is responsible for the complaint, without pursuing the matter further.

The two most frequently prescribed forms of the hormone which have been used in premenstrual syndrome therapy have been straightforward progesterone, and dydrogesterone. Apart from the question of their efficacy in treating this complaint, the use of steroids (hormones) is not appropriate to all patients, and there is a five to ten per cent incidence of minor side-effects.[2]

In this connection, you may think of the side-effects which you have heard attributed to the Pill. Most of the side-effects of oral contraceptives are due to the oestrogen they contain rather than to their progesterone content, but the latter still accounts for a number of unpleasant symptoms when given to women who are especially susceptible to them.

Jackie Gill was a patient of mine, and came to see me when the progesterone pessary I had prescribed for her seemed to have drawbacks. This was several years ago, before the recent discoveries discussed later in this book were made, and progesterone therapy was one of the standard forms of treatment for premenstrual symptoms.

Jackie was a twenty-three-year-old secretary, unmarried, and healthy apart from the swollen, painful breasts and great tension which she experienced for four or five days every month before her period was due to start. She was not taking any other form of medication when I suggested that she try the pessaries (*Cyclogest*) to see whether they would improve her symptoms.

After trying them for two months, she came back to see me. 'My breasts are far less tender, Doctor, and I don't seem nearly as snappy as I used to be when I'm waiting for "the curse" to start – but I have been feeling awfully apathetic, depressed and tired. Do you think this is just due to the time of the month, or could it be anything to do with those pessaries you gave me?'

This rang a warning bell with me at once, because side-effects associated with the use of progesterone compounds include fatigue, lethargy, depression and a lack of initiative, i.e. inertia. Jackie's lethargy had been fairly troublesome, and so we had to discontinue the treatment.[3]

Another theory about the cause of the premenstrual syndrome is that it is due to excessively high levels of oestrogen in the blood, which, it is said, are capable of inducing the depressive symptoms and the mental disturbance in particular. The reason that you may get depressed if your oestrogen output is greater than that of many other women is that the oestrogen can interfere with the chemical mechanism involving vitamin B_6 (pyridoxine). This is known as the 'anti-depression vitamin', because it controls the production of a compound called serotonin. Serotonin is essential for brain and nerve function and an inadequate supply causes depression.

A link between large amounts of oestrogen in the bloodstream and premenstrual depression was first suspected when the similarity was noticed between the depression of the premenstrual syndrome and the depression a number of women experience when they are on the Pill. The depression associated with the contraceptive Pill is known to be due to the synthetic oestrogen that it contains.

One trial carried out at St Mary's Hospital, London, involved a group of thirty-nine women suffering from depression as a result of taking the Pill. Nineteen of these women were found to be lacking in vitamin B$_6$, and every one of these, when treated with forty milligrams of the vitamin daily, responded by losing all signs of depression. No improvement was detected in the remaining twenty women with normal vitamin B$_6$ levels, despite prolonged treatment with the vitamin.[4]

Supplementing the diet with pyridoxine is now an established approach to treating the premenstrual syndrome, and this vitamin can have a beneficial effect on a number of the symptoms associated with it. Besides depression, fluid retention is lessened and patients notice in particular that their fingers and ankles are less swollen.

Penny Lloyd, a forty-year-old landscape gardener, was particularly affected by swollen fingers. As her job involved a lot of outdoor work she tended to use gardening gloves a great deal, particularly during the winter. These had to be quite closely fitting because she went from greenhouse to greenhouse for several hours each morning, where she worked with small, delicate plants and used correspondingly delicate tools for the task.

Her fingers swelled up so much in the week before her period started that she found it impossible to get her gloves on. In fact she came to see me to get something for her chilblains which were an inevitable result of going gloveless. She mentioned how her hands swelled up, but she had not heard of this happening premenstrually and had thought it was due to a chemical she had been using with her plant work. I started her on pyridoxine at a rate of fifty milligrams daily to be taken every day for ten days before her period started each month – and this satisfactorily controlled the tendency to swell.

Doses as high as five hundred milligrams per day have to be prescribed for some women before they respond satisfactorily.

Another hormone – prolactin – has also been indicted as a cause of premenstrual symptoms. It is produced by the pituitary gland and it affects the amounts of oestrogen and progesterone that are produced during each cycle. Too much prolactin upsets the delicately balanced mechanism governing the production of these two hormones, and some of the effects of too little progesterone or too much oestrogen, are felt. Prolactin really comes into its own after you have had a baby, because its most important function is to stimulate the breasts to produce milk. But it is being produced all the time by the pituitary, and large amounts of it can affect breast tissue during the premenstrual phase of your cycle, making the breasts enlarged, tense, swollen and very tender. A number of women suffering from the premenstrual syndrome are found to have higher than normal levels of prolactin in their blood. In them, the symptoms respond well to a drug called bromocriptine which suppresses the secretion of prolactin by the pituitary gland.

The majority of women suffering from the premenstrual syndrome who have been studied, however, have normal levels of prolactin. So while high levels of this hormone may be implicated in a number of cases of the premenstrual syndrome, as evidenced by the benefit they receive when prolactin secretion is suppressed, it is certainly not the final and complete answer to the cause of the illness.

Jill Majors, aged thirty, and a talented window-dresser, was disappointed by her experience of bromocriptine – although in her case this was not due to the drug's inefficiency, but to a faulty laboratory result.

Some years ago I treated her with progesterone for premenstrual illness but she had to discontinue the therapy as it did not suit her. I arranged for a blood test at the local hospital and her prolactin level was reported as being unusually high. I checked the result with the chief technician, who assured me that their brand new apparatus for making this difficult measurement was working perfectly and that the result I had been sent was correct.

I prescribed bromocriptine for Jill and it had no effect whatsoever upon her mood swings, depression and sore, enlarged breasts. I discontinued the treatment after I heard from my partner that the hospital had sent out a report stating that, for the first three weeks of using their new machinery, they had unwittingly been sending out excessively high results to all the local GPs who had requested blood tests to be performed by it!

At the start of this chapter, I mentioned that it is now thought that the underlying cause of the premenstrual syndrome is a deficiency in the body of essential fatty acids (EFAs); and that this deficiency can produce the same effect in women as a raised prolactin level can, because when EFAs are in short supply the body is abnormally sensitive to ordinary levels of this hormone.

Put another way, higher than normal levels of the pituitary hormone prolactin produce symptoms of the premenstrual syndrome in a number of women who suffer from this illness. But there are many premenstrual syndrome sufferers who, when their prolactin levels are measured, are found to have normal levels of this hormone in their blood. There is now evidence showing that being deficient in EFAs, *has the same effect* on a woman as a considerably raised prolactin level has, i.e. it can produce disturbances in her metabolism attributable to oestrogen and progesterone imbalance. The prolactin level itself is normal; and so, often, are the measured levels of oestrogen and progesterone. But because the body is lacking in EFAs, it is hypersensitive to the normal level of prolactin which is present. Instead of actually having too much prolactin, the affected woman has too few EFAs – but with respect to premenstrual symptoms this amounts to the same thing.

Where does the usefulness of pyridoxine, vitamin B_6, fit into all this? Pyridoxine increases the efficiency with which the body tissues make use of EFAs. So, for a person who is lacking the right amount of essential fatty acids, taking a supplement of pyridoxine will enable her to utilize the supply of EFAs that is available to her, to the best possible advantage.

As a corollary of this, it is now known that hormonal imbalance can increase the requirement for pyridoxine to much greater than normal. So while the measurement of your pyridoxine level could be useful if you really had a very low level of this vitamin in your bloodstream, what the reading would not show would be the possible case of your having a 'normal' reading which was, in fact, far too low for your own personal requirements.

This explains why many women are helped considerably by taking pyridoxine supplements when they do not appear to be actually deficient in this vitamin. One could call into question the twenty women in the St Mary's Hospital trial, mentioned earlier in this chapter, who had Pill-induced depression but no apparent pyridoxine deficiency and who were *not* helped by pyridoxine supplements, in contrast to the other nineteen women who *did* have low vitamin levels and who were helped by taking pyridoxine. The probable explanation for this is that, for the twenty women concerned, their own particular pyridoxine levels were sufficient for their own particular requirements.

This in fact emphasizes the truth of the statement that each and every woman has her own special premenstrual (and hormonal) profile and her own particular needs with respect to treatment. Hormonal imbalance plays a major role in the various manifestations of the premenstrual syndrome; but it now seems that a widespread lack of essential fatty acids is the probable common factor in the causation of premenstrual illness.

Now we know what the premenstrual syndrome is and a little about why it occurs, the next essential is to decide whether or not you are suffering from it.

[1] Sampson, G.A. 'The Premenstrual Syndrome', *British Journal of Psychiatry* 135 (1979), pp.209-215.

[2] Kerr, G. D; Day, J. B; Munday, M. R; Brush, M. G; Watson, M. and Taylor, R. W., 'Dydrogesterone in the treatment of the premenstrual syndrome', *Practitioner* 224 (1980), pp.852-855.

[3] Mervyn, L. *The B Vitamins* (Thorsons Publishers, 1981).

[4] Murad, F. and Gilman, A. G. 'Estrogens and Progestins' in *The Pharmacological Basis of Theraputics* (ed. L. S. Goodman and A. Gilman, Macmillan Publishing Co. Inc., New York, 1975).

5

Do I Suffer From It?

Do you get depressed? Are your breasts sometimes tender and sore? Do you crave for certain kinds of food, snap at your husband, feel like shooting your boss and put on weight easily?

You may be suffering from the premenstrual syndrome. On the other hand, all the physical and psychological features listed above are extremely common and it is perfectly possible to suffer from all of them, without their constituting premenstrual illness. The definition of the condition is all-important, so it is worth restating it here:

> The premenstrual syndrome is a group of physical and mental changes which begin anything from two to fourteen days before menstruation, and which are relieved almost immediately the period starts.

No doctor would diagnose the premenstrual syndrome on the strength of a single set of symptoms, i.e. if a woman visits his surgery and complains of feeling tense and depressed, and of having tender, enlarged breasts, nausea, weight gain and a bad headache. Her period may be due to start at any moment and the symptoms strongly suggest the premenstrual syndrome, but in order to state with certainty that a woman is suffering from this illness, the doctor must be sure that her symptoms recur on a regular monthly basis.

Take another look at the symptoms, which are listed in an easy-to-check form below, and make a mental note of the ones which affect you.

Physical symptoms
Weight gain
Swelling (abdomen, fingers, legs, ankles)
Feeling of bloatedness
Breast discomfort (enlargement, tenderness, heaviness, generalized 'lumpiness')
Headaches
Migraine attacks
Muscular aches and pains, stiffness
Congestive dysmenorrhoea
Low urine output
Skin changes, including blotches, acne, whiteheads, unexplained bruising
Changes in appetite (either loss of appetite, or desire to eat a great deal of fattening foods)
Sleep changes (either sleeping poorly, or sleeping a great deal more than usual)
Clumsiness and an increased proneness to accidents
Diminished exercise tolerance, i.e. an abnormal degree of fatigue in relation to physical exertion
Painful eyes
Nasal stuffiness
Allergic reactions
If asthmatic or epileptic, an increased tendency to attacks
Nausea, faintness

Psychological symptoms
Tension
Irritability
Depression, including lack of confidence and notions of unworthiness

Lethargy
Reduced power of concentration
Poor memory
Tendency to aggressiveness and/or physical violence
Poor emotional control
Illogical emotional reactions
Lowered efficiency, especially for solving mental problems
Low or absent sex drive
Very strong urges to overeat, unrelated to appetite
Tendency to drink too much alcohol
Increased tendency to take tablets, medicine, etc.

It may be obvious to you that you are suffering from the premenstrual syndrome because you have clear-cut symptoms that coincide with the checklist and recur at regular intervals during the premenstrual phase of your cycles.

For many women, however, the answer may be less obvious, particularly for women to whom the concept of the premenstrual syndrome is new. Even if you keep a diary and note the dates on which you feel unwell, you still have to leaf through it time and time again, remembering to fill in the symptoms whenever they occur, and it is less easy to obtain an overall picture of recurrent complaints from diary entries than it is if you enter the type of complaint and when it happens, on a properly designed chart.

One example of such a chart, completed by a sufferer from premenstrual tension, is given in Figure 1, while Figure 2 shows the sort of picture obtained when a non-sufferer fills her symptoms in, i.e. a woman who periodically gets depression, bouts of compulsive eating, weight gain and irritability which are not in fact due to the premenstrual syndrome.

Notice how the symptoms on the first chart, which was filled in by Jane Winter, the medical student discussed in Chapter 4, are grouped together during the days when she is expecting her period, and cease pretty well as soon as menstruation begins. Notice, too, how the symptoms shown on the next menstrual chart are scattered at random, and bear no relation to the woman's premenstrual phase. They are not relieved when she starts to bleed, and they occur as often during the immediate post-menstrual phase (when premenstrual syndrome sufferers are at their best) as they do at other times.

Figure 1: Premenstrual Chart 1

	September	October	November	December
1		U↓	U↓ W L	U↓ W L B
2		U↓ W L	U↓ W L	U↓ W L B
3		U↓ W L	U↓ W L	U↓ W L B
4	U↓	U↓ W L	U↓ W L	U↓ W L B
5	U↓ W L	U↓ W L	U↓ W L	U↓ W L B
6	U↓ W L	U↓ W L	U↓ W L B	P U↑
7	U↓ W L	U↓ W L B	U↓ W L B	P
8	U↓ W L	U↓ W L B	P U↑	P
9	U↓ W L	U↓ W L B	P U↑	P
10	U↓ W L	U↓ W L B	P	
11	U↓ W L B	P U↓ W	P	
12	U↓ W L B	P U↑	P	
13	U↓ W L B	P U↑		
14	P U↑	P		
15	P	P		
16	P			
17	P			
18	P			
19				
20				
21				
22				
23				
24				
25				
26				
27				
28				
29			U↓ W L	
30			U↓ W L	
31				

W = weight gain	B = tender breasts
I = irritability	D = depression
P = period days	V = violent tendencies
U↓ = urine output less than usual	L = lethargy
U↑ = urine output more than usual	C = cravings for food/drink

Reproduced by kind permission of St. Thomas' Hospital, London.

Figure 2: Premenstrual Chart 2

	September	October	November	December
1		P	P	
2		P	P	
3		P		
4		P		
5		P		
6				
7				
8				
9	D C			D
10	D C I		I	
11	D C W I		I	D C
12	D C W I		C I	
13			C I W	
14				I
15				
16				
17				
18				
19				
20				
21				D C
22				D C W
23				P D C
24				P D C W
25		D	P	P D C W
26		D C	P	P D C W
27		D C	P	P
28		P D C W I	P	P
29		P D C W I	P	P I
30	P	P D C W I		I
31		P D C W I		I

W	= weight gain		B	= tender breasts
I	= irritability		V	= violent tendencies
P	= period days		D	= depression
U↓	= urine output less than usual		L	= lethargy
U↑	= urine output more than usual		C	= cravings for food/drink

Reproduced by kind permission of St. Thomas' Hospital, London.

Using these as a guide, draw up your own chart and fill it in over a period of at least two consecutive months – preferably more – and then compare your chart with the two given. Enter your symptoms, opposite the day on which they occur, using the first letter of the symptom as a symbol, e.g. I for irritability, and W for weight gain. It is a good idea to enter the symptoms using one colour (perhaps green), and save another colour (red) for the letter P to indicate the days on which you have your period. It is then easy to see at a glance, whether you have the typical pattern of symptoms that indicates premenstrual illness, or whether they occur at random as in the second chart.

I always represent a fall in usual urine output per day, by a U followed by a downward-pointing arrow, and an increased urinary output by a U and an upward-pointing arrow. You should find that, within a few hours of your period starting, you are passing larger amounts of urine than usual – certainly larger than you have been passing since your premenstrual symptoms started. This is the sign that your tissues are getting rid of the excessive amounts of fluid they have been retaining, and should make you decidedly cheerful as the physical and psychological miseries caused by fluid retention are in the process of disappearing. Diminished urine excretion, followed in the way I have described by an increased output, are very important symptoms and should not be ignored; so fill in any changes you notice in this respect on your chart, as soon as they become apparent.

Your menstrual period, as shown on your chart, should be followed by a number of completely symptom-free days, and you will very likely find that your premenstrual symptoms restart at the same point in your cycle every month. For instance, counting the day your period starts as day one, your symptoms should fade and disappear over days one and two and you should be consistently symptom-free until, say, day sixteen of your monthly cycle, when your symptoms start to reappear.

A further value of this chart is that you become aware of the day in your monthly cycle on which you can expect to feel premenstrual. Not only does this enable you to take precautions to avoid extra stress on this and subsequent days; it also means that, using the kind of treatment I shall be discussing later on, you can start treatment a couple of days in advance, and in this way stand an excellent chance of avoiding the symptoms altogether.

The other kind of chart which will help you is the symptom score chart, given in Figure 3. This was prepared at St Thomas' Hospital, London, where there is a major premenstrual syndrome centre, and its object is to indicate the severity of your symptoms. Use it by entering, on of the form, the day of your cycle on which the various symptoms start and the day on which they end, for example, day twenty-five of one cycle, and day two of the following one.

Remember that day one is always the day on which you start to bleed. Indicate the severity of your symptoms by the number of ticks which you place opposite each one on the chart – one for mild, two for moderate and three for severe.

I have mentioned a number of symptoms that do not appear on this chart which, for the sake of convenience, is necessarily limited in size. In the column marked 'Other symptoms' you can fill in one that bothers you a lot – and enter an extra column or two on the form for others if necessary.

It is easier first to use the menstrual chart and then to use the symptom score chart. You can then see at a glance which your 'start' and 'end' dates are. Fill in the charts carefully for at least two consecutive months and, if you wish, see your doctor. This is always advisable if you are unduly bothered about a particular symptom, and are not certain whether it fits into the premenstrual syndrome or whether it is an independent trouble.

Your doctor may be very sympathetic towards you as an premenstrual syndrome sufferer or he may not. This book will set you on the right road towards self-help and enable you to overcome the illness, but your doctor is invaluable in that he is in a position to diagnose your complaint first-hand – and either reassure you that your illness is premenstrual or that you need further investigations.

Always go to your doctor if you suffer from any of the following: persistent breast lump(s), that is, a lump or area of tense breast tissue that remains with you constantly and does not come and go with your premenstrual phases; migraine or other troublesome headaches that continue to incapacitate you despite the treatment advocated in this book; a copious, smelly, vaginal discharge before, during or after your period; severe depression

Figure 3: Symptom Score Chart

Symptom	Day of Cycle (Start) (Finish)		Severity of symptoms
Weight gain			
Swellings			
Breast discomfort			
Headaches			
Muscular aches			
Congestive dysmenorrhoea			
Low urine output			
Appetite changes			
Sleep changes			
Poor co-ordination			
Other physical symptoms			
Tension/irritability			
Depression			
Lethargy			
Poor concentration			
Aggressive tendencies			
Low or absent sex drive			
Food craving			
Alcohol craving			
Need for isolation			
Poor emotional control			
Other psychological symptoms			

Reproduced by kind permission of St Thomas' Hospital, London.

that is not relieved by premenstrual remedies; anything else whatsoever that really bothers you and which you would like to have sorted out.

The next chapter will make suggestions about how best to cope with premenstrual symptoms and your job at the same time.

6

The Premenstrual Syndrome: At Work

In this and the following two chapters, we will look at the best ways of coping with the problem of the premenstrual syndrome: firstly, if you go to work; secondly, at home; and thirdly, at school.

But there is one piece of advice that pertains, regardless of the environment in which you find yourself: do not just put up with your troubles. There is no virtue whatever in that type of suffering and there is no need for it now that help is at hand. If you suffer badly from premenstrual illness, your attempts to 'grin and bear it' may, if the day goes badly, become a macabre caricature and metamorphose into the 'risus sardonicus' – sardonic grin – of real suffering.

No one will thank you for your martyrdom, least of all those whom you think should be most grateful for your heroic efforts. So read on, and find out how to make life much easier for yourself when female biology gives you a lot to contend with.

You may well protest that you want to read about the revolutionary new treatment that is available, and so why am I writing three chapters about how to cope with the problem, thereby suggesting that you will continue to suffer from it. Personally, I do not have a great deal of faith in 'wonder drugs' and am generally pretty sceptical about 'miracle cures'. The new dietary approach developed from the discovery of essential fatty acid deficiency already mentioned, is achieving a very high success rate in correcting the imbalance which is responsible for the premenstrual syndrome. And you may well read about it, start taking it and never have another day of trouble.

On the other hand, there is no one compound in the world which can be guaranteed immediately to clear up every single symptom of a given illness in every single person who suffers from it. Again, you may have to wait until you have an opportunity to go and buy the product, or find yourself away on holiday abroad, faced with the symptoms and with no remedy at hand; or you might, in any case, simply wish to amass as much advice as possible from as many sources as you have access to, in order to get maximum help in dealing with very difficult days.

Here, then, are suggestions for coping with a day at work during the premenstrual syndrome; I have compiled the details from hundreds of conversations with premenstrual sufferers who have had to devise ways of maintaining their efficiency even though they may feel very off-colour. I must stress at this point that I do not consider every woman who suffers from some degree of the premenstrual syndrome to be a partial or even a potential invalid. But coping adequately with a responsible job (and every job you can think of confers a certain amount of responsibility); running a house and looking after children; or getting through a demanding day at school or college, can be very tough, especially if you feel fat, unattractive, lethargic and clumsy – and have a bad headache into the bargain!

The secret of success, of swimming rather than sinking, is organization – or, as it often turns out, reorganization. The object is to give yourself maximum freedom from stress, and to avoid the obvious pitfalls and obstacles, while still allowing you to do your fair share. Putting yourself in a position in which you can be criticized for shirking, in order to give yourself an easy time, is only adding to your problems.

Let's begin when you wake up in the morning feeling decidedly premenstrual. If you feel *too* bad – stay in bed! By this I do not mean, 'ask your doctor for a sick note every time you get a symptom of the illness', when you could cope perfectly well with a little self-help and forethought. And neither do I mean you to give in to an urge that commonly afflicts sufferers then, which is to pull the duvet over your head and lie there hoping the world will go away! I am referring to the occasions when you have a severe migraine, nausea and dizziness, or really painful congestive dysmenorrhoea. Anything, in fact, which will inevitably make your day, and other people's, thoroughly miserable.

If you have a severe headache or migraine, you are obviously unfit to drive and will only make matters worse by travelling on rush-hour public transport. If you feel nauseous and dizzy, then you are a liability anywhere but in your own bathroom; and if you have severe congestive pelvic pain, you will sound, look and act exactly like a wet week, for that is just how you will feel.

So with any of these symptoms stay in bed, have a cup of weak tea and a couple of aspirin, and make an appointment to see your doctor as soon as possible.

But let's suppose you are going to work. Don't skip breakfast. I used to do this as a teenager and a medical student but felt decidedly stupid after fainting in the train on the way to the hospital one morning and reporting at the students' sick bay – and having to admit to the staff doctor that I hadn't taken the simple precaution of eating a slice of toast and taking a drink before leaving home.

You may lose your appetite altogether when premenstrual, but at the very least do swallow some freshly-squeezed grapefruit or orange juice, with a little added glucose or honey, and half a slice of wholemeal bread, lightly toasted and with a scraping of butter or Marmite. Drink weak tea or milky coffee or, better still, a glass of mineral water. You will not then be adding the risk of hypoglycaemia (low blood sugar) to your problems halfway through the morning.

If you can face getting up ten minutes earlier on premenstrual mornings, you can put this bonus of extra time to very good advantage. Use it to make yourself look as nice as possible. When you have the handicaps of acne, a protruding stomach, thick ankles and perhaps the involuntary frown of a tension headache, you do not want to add to your troubles by staying in bed until the least possible moment and going out breakfastless and in crumpled old clothes that you normally wear for bathing the dog – plus no make-up and with your hair standing on end.

Splash cold water on your face to get your skin glowing, or at least moisten your skin with a pleasant-smelling cleansing and toning lotion on a cotton-wool pad, and follow this with a light make-up base, your favourite lipstick and a little eyeshadow, not forgetting to use a blemish pencil to disguise spots and blotchy areas.

Then, before you get dressed, fling off your dressing gown, stand in front of the window and do the following exercise, which will take about two minutes at the outside and really will improve the way you feel. Stand upright, tall as you can, arms at your sides. Breathe in slowly and deeply, until your lungs are as full as possible. Hold this for a count of three and then expel the air. Repeat twice, and then follow this by making large circles with your arms, bringing them up from in front of you to either side of your head so that your upper arms just brush your ears. Swing them backwards behind you as far as you can reach, so that the muscles in your shoulders, neck and upper arms are stretched fully without being strained. Do this twice more. Finally, with your feet pointing forward and about eighteen inches apart, bend down and touch your toes – or try to!

This exercise is not designed to help you to lose weight. Its object is to tone up your muscles, step up your metabolic rate, improve your overall sense of well-being, and actually make you *feel* thinner! It may be said, at this point, that because your body tends to retain water premenstrually and because this fluid retention is responsible for many of the symptoms of the premenstrual syndrome, it is a good idea to reduce your fluid intake below your normal amount, as soon as you are aware that your urine output is less than usual. It is impossible to give you an actual volume to cut down to; we all have different fluid needs, depending to a certain extent on the type of activity in which we are engaged, and the temperature in which we spend most of our time. Don't feel uncomfortably thirsty and deny yourself a drink. But avoid drinking unnecessarily and, at the same time, take as little salt as you can. Sodium chloride (common salt) tends to keep fluid in the body, which you are anxious to avoid. So use very little salt in cooking and don't add any to your food. Also avoid salty snacks such as peanuts, crisps and Twiglets. This is a sound health measure anyway, as there is plenty of evidence that large amounts of salt are associated with a high blood pressure and a number of heart conditions.

Get your day off to a good start by making certain that you look as attractive as the other people with whom you work. If you don't wear a uniform, then choose items of clothes that look good, and which are both comfortable and practical. Many women tend to perspire more freely during their premenstrual phase and, with that fact in mind, cotton underwear is both hygienic and easy to wear. If your breasts enlarge and feel swollen and tender, rather than go braless buy a bra one size or one fitting larger than you usually need, in your favourite brand, and keep as your 'special' bra for just such occasions.

You'll never feel at your best if you look dowdy. It's of paramount importance to give yourself every advantage at this time – keep a special outfit or two set aside for wearing on premenstrual syndrome days. I don't mean a size twenty tent-dress – unless, of course, you happen to be a size twenty and look good in tent-dresses! Select something loose, comfortable and smart, in a colour that is serene and calm, rather than aggressive, dramatic or visually violent. Try cream, grey, green or soft blue, in preference to purple, orange or scarlet. And try to avoid black, it's far too funereal.

The best ways of travelling to work if you are suffering from premenstrual symptoms are either to walk, if it is not too far, or to obtain a lift. Cycling, riding a motor-bike, or driving are not choice means of transport at a time when you are very likely to be slow and clumsy, and accident-prone. See if you can organize a lift for yourself, perhaps by offering a reciprocal lift to a friend on other days of the month.

If neither walking nor being driven is possible, and you are obliged to travel by public transport, try to remember the night before to get everything ready for your departure in the morning. There is no worse start to a day than hunting desperately for a set of notes, your keys or some loose change. And do remember to have a raincoat and umbrella at the ready – on 'bad' days it is so often raining into the bargain!

If you cannot avoid driving, make sure that the car has enough petrol and oil, decent tyres and a live battery. And that it can be depended upon to start, even on cold mornings. If you are stuck with a non-starter, skip it and ring for a mini-cab. Better a few pounds less in your account to spend on vodka and tights than a respectable bank balance and a car that ends up as a write-off, because in your understandable rage at its tardiness in starting you have wrapped it round a lamp-post!

Having got to work, whatever you do for a living – be it in an office, factory, hotel, school or hospital – the place is bound to be a positive minefield teeming with irritants and stress factors that can fret, annoy or simply upset you when your nerves are very much on edge. Many jobs are harder on individuals now that redundancy is rife, and the strain on personnel is multiplied by a factor of several. So approach work hazards by making a list in advance of the pitfalls you are likely to encounter and plan some counter-measures to overcome them.

If your desk is normally tidy – that's fine! If it generally resembles a compost heap, i.e. it contains some good things of potentially great value but bears to the unpractised eye a close resemblance to a rubbish tip, then start excavating the various strata now and throw away everything that is useless. Better the constant though minor fag of keeping your desk tidy, where everything can be found at a glance or at the swish-open of a drawer, than the usual fuss and flap which is magnified many times on a premenstrual day, of having to search for a particular document, set of notes, Biro or Tipp-Ex bottle.

Keep, in a drawer of your desk, a number of emergency measures, or what I call a premenstrual first-aid kit. The true dressing of the day's wounds, should you suffer any, can take place with full examination of their severity and depth, at home later on, in the comfort and security of your love nest or family. I'll tell you how to go about that too, later on. But in the meantime, see that your private drawer contains some or all of the following – depending on your own special needs.

Firstly, a pair of sun-glasses: these have a number of uses and many women find them indispensable. If you suffer from irrational emotions and suddenly develop an intense if transitory hatred for your boss or a rapturous passion for Head of Accounts, wearing dark glasses allows you to smoulder, glower and/or entice the object of your aroused emotions without the least harm or embarrassment resulting from the intensity of your gaze. Additionally, dark glasses can make you look sexy and interesting, never a bad thing when you are feeling the reverse. And if someone does upset you, and you lose your temper and have a good cry about it in the Ladies, you can explain airily as you emerge from your hideout, that you are wearing dark glasses because you have a headache. There will be no fear of the signs of your misery being apparent in the form of red eyes.

Levity aside, this brings me to the most important use you are likely to find for your sun-glasses. If you are prone either to tension headaches or to migraine attacks, you will find that these can be very much aggravated by fluorescent lighting. So buy as good a pair of sun-glasses as you can afford and keep them in your desk. You'll find them invaluable.

Other items I would recommend for your premenstrual first-aid kit include: tissues; some soluble aspirin or another pain-killer of your choice, for the headache or stomach-ache you cannot ward off; some glucose sweets to suck if you have hunger pangs; a set of worry beads, obtainable from Indian markets and similar shops in this country, and marvellous for dispelling tension – also a more attractive habit than nail-biting or smoking; a spare note pad and Biro for the things you think you are bound to forget, such as phone messages, family matters you remember during the day, etc.; and a couple of Tampax or disposable towels just in case your period should arrive early.

Do you suffer from appetite changes or food/drink cravings due to the premenstrual syndrome? If you simply go off food entirely for a few days but eat normally during the rest of your cycle, you are probably well adjusted to the situation and are able to keep your weight stable by eating rather more than usual once your period has started to compensate for the days when you cannot face a thing to eat.

Some women, however, have rather longer premenstrual phases than the relatively brief 'three or four days'. As we have seen, symptoms of the premenstrual syndrome can start as early in the cycle as fourteen days before the next period is due – and if you are anorexic (the technical term for loss of appetite) for as long as that, you may have some difficulty in maintaining a stable weight balance. This is the time to treat yourself to a special delicacy or two which you may not normally think of buying for yourself, and which would be far too exotic or expensive for an ordinary worktime lunch. Go out and buy them before your premenstrual phase starts and take them to work to brighten up your lunch hour. This is not an ordinary time and you need extra pampering – so if you would find it impossible to swallow a round of sandwiches and a beer, or something from the canteen, try a thin slice of Parma ham and some chilled ripe melon, or a choice piece of ripe Camembert with a small bunch of hothouse grapes, or a few fresh prawns and half a ripe avocado.

If even these leave you untouched and untempted, could you face a cup of hot, fresh coffee and a piece of your favourite Swiss milk chocolate? Normally I strongly advocate eating only organically grown wholefoods – but this preference can be set aside for the moment in order to persuade you to eat at least *something* during the day, even when your appetite is very poor.

If your appetite disturbance goes the other way and you are unable to leave food alone, keep something safe, calorie-wise, to eat when your stomach is at its most demanding, to try to avoid buying fattening junk-food snacks to fill you up instead. Avoid like the plague foods such as chocolate, biscuits, ice-cream, chips and thick sandwiches containing lots of butter or margarine and great slabs of cream cheese, fat meat or peanut butter mixed with honey. It's amazing what the demon inside you, whom you normally control so well, will insist on having when your higher rational centres temporarily lose control.

Take with you a delicious, filling but not fattening lunch, and keep a few snacks with you in case of an emergency. Wrap up some freshly-washed celery in greaseproof paper, and add some radishes, spring onions, small tomatoes and watercress to eat as well. Take a tub of yogurt, some cottage cheese and an apple, pear or peach. If you yearn unceasingly for something sweet, rich-tasting and chewable, I recommend a fruit and nut bar from a health-food shop. Made with delicious items such as dried apricots, figs and dates, they are sweetened with honey or brown sugar only, and contain a variety of other goodies such as toasted hazelnuts, sesame seeds, sunflower seeds, sultanas and raisins. They certainly are not junk food. But they satisfy the intense cravings that can strike you and ruin your diet month after month.

Keep several such bars in your first-aid drawer, and eat one as and when you most need it.

Now, with respect to work itself: if you are in a position to organize your own working day, see that your days are at their least demanding during your premenstrual phase. Avoid important meetings if you possibly can, choosing dates for them when you are likely to be at your best, i.e. straight after your period is over. Try instead to arrange your schedule so that, on difficult days, your work is of the type you can do at your own pace, and preferably by yourself. Better still, get a bit ahead of your work schedule during your good phase, so that you can afford to take things just that little bit more easily when you are premenstrual.

There is nothing wrong in this. You are not mollycoddling yourself, cheating your employer or skiving off so that your colleagues are lumbered with more than their fair share. Of course you cannot run your life and fashion the control of a demanding job according to your premenstrual phases only. But it is an indisputable, if regrettable, fact that, if you suffer from premenstrual syndrome, you are likely to work less efficiently for a few days each month, and that your poorer powers of concentration and reduced memory ability will inevitably affect your overall efficiency. So if you can work extra diligently before your premenstrual phase is due to start – and you will know exactly when to expect it from your menstrual chart – then it makes sense to go easy on yourself when possible. You will, after all, have earned the right by your forethought.

Furthermore, make sure that you spend your lunch-hour the way that suits *you* during the period of time we are discussing. If you feel nervy, and perhaps a bit 'shut in' by the building in which you work, go out and stretch your legs for a bit. But choose, as your objective, a walk in the fresh air rather than a duty trip round the supermarket or into the nearest department store for a birthday present or to accompany your friend who wants to buy a new dress. This would only be swopping one set of central heating and fluorescent lighting for another. Refuse nicely to spend any dutiful lunch-hours when you have premenstrual illness. If something is needed for the evening meal, ask your partner to get it on the way home, or use an alternative recipe. Present buying can be easily planned to fit into a weekend instead of being crammed into a brief lunch-hour. And if your dress sense is invaluable to your friend, ask her to wait till you feel more like going shopping with her.

Also – except for a real emergency – avoid working lunch-hours. It happens to us all sometimes, and when it is inevitable, make the best of it and try not to grumble. But if you are under the weather that is all the more reason to have your lunch-time to please yourself in, so do your best to see that you get it. Any irritability the morning may have provoked can be disposed of much more satisfactorily by means of a brisk walk around the park and sitting for half an hour in the sunshine on a quiet bench. Even this little bit of contact with nature can make you feel like humming a tune as you return when your hour is up. A complicated telephone call to Düsseldorf, searching for a client's specifications which you have lost, or going through yesterday's correspondence, do nothing for pent-up frustration and a nagging headache.

The same basic principles apply if you work in a school, hospital, library, airport or department store. Provide yourself with a change of scenery and some fresh air if you feel jumpy and tense; or if you feel just plain tired and achey, make for the rest-room, staff sitting-room or whatever facilities are provided. Even the privacy of your own desk can give you a certain amount of security if you are feeling vulnerable and anti-social. Just make certain that you allow yourself a little bit of selfishness during your working day – you'll cope much better, and for longer, if you do look after yourself in this way.

When you get a few moments to yourself – even if you have to visit the Ladies to achieve this end – 'switch off' for a little, rest . . . and relax. . . . Think of the Zen Buddhist principle of refusing to fight your adversaries and environment but flowing with the tide of life instead. Let tension seep out of you, and picture in your mind's eye, the starry heavens as you have seen them on a clear, silent, cold night. Project yourself upwards until you are up there among the stars – then look down, and see how infinitesimal the planet Earth is; how microscopic the seas, oceans and continents; the people, too tiny to imagine. Just how important is your own problem in all the wondrous immensity of the Universe?

Come slowly back to Earth when you're ready, take a few deep breaths, and your relaxed state of repose should, with luck, remain with you for the rest of the day.

By the same token, make sure you do your fair share of unpopular jobs and extra work, and make sure in an unobtrusive way that other people are aware that you do your fair share! Just avoid volunteering for overtime duties or heavy physical work during the week before your period is due. Take minimum work home with you, too. You probably wouldn't do it anyway, and you need the evening to recuperate and relax.

Once home for the evening, discard your workaday image and pamper yourself. If you live alone, you have all the opportunity in the world for this, so make the most of it, for the chances are that you may well be sharing your life with someone else soon, and the chance to be utterly selfish will be a little diminished! The best thing to do is – whatever you most feel like doing! Go straight to bed with a drink and a plate of sandwiches or fruit, and watch television, play a screen game, look at a favourite old movie if you own a video – or get out of bed and dance yourself to a standstill to your favourite music, if you've a mind to. Let yourself go, relax and enjoy your evening. Or, if you are dog tired, fall into a warm bath, take the phone off the hook and flake out. The choice is entirely yours!

If you have a husband or lover and family, get them to cherish you particularly tenderly during your premenstrual syndrome. There is an art in getting people to do this, and it is straightforward and easy to apply once you know the secret. Firstly, confide in them or, at least, in those who are old enough to understand, and it's surprising how much young children can comprehend if you approach them in the right way. Explain, in words to suit each family member, what the premenstrual syndrome is, and that you suffer from it, and that you are / will be having treatment for it. Say you realize that you are difficult to live with during that time and would really appreciate their co-operation during that time of the month. It is surprising how often apparently selfish and insensitive people will rally round when given the courtesy of an explanation and their compliance is specially requested. Better still, give them this book to read; they will be in no doubt then that your problem is a real one, and that you need all the help you can get.

Secondly, be ready and willing to reciprocate. Every single one of us has difficulties with which to contend, and feels 'under the weather' at certain times. It is also possible, without being premenstrual, to feel fat, unattractive, stupid and inadequate – and to suffer from depression, headaches and tension. The chief difference is that the symptoms in other people are unlikely to be due to a deficiency of essential fatty acids affecting them through the medium of their hormonal systems, and because they are not cyclical they are far less predictable. So ask your husband, parents or children to let you know when a difficult day is going to come up at work or at school – or when they just wake up and feel in their bones that it is going to be a 'bad' day. Be gentle and understanding, and especially loving when they come in, in the evening. Run a bath for them, plan something they are particularly fond of for supper and do some small thing you know they'll notice and like, such as performing their ironing task, buying them a small gift, or leaving a few flowers in a teenage daughter's bedroom. If you cringe at the thought of being so obvious and banal – do it anyway! Bravado and the sought-after macho image account for a great deal of overtough he-men, many of whom have hearts of gold if you know how to recognize the often rather base exterior metal!

Communication and a willingness to meet other people halfway is the name of the game with respect to your family at home. But while on this theme – however well you know the people with whom you work, I would be strongly disinclined to announce to all and sundry at the office that you are suffering from the premenstrual syndrome. This has absolutely nothing whatever to do with the idea that sex and related subjects are 'not nice' discussion topics: the more we know about our complaints, the sooner medical science will find a solution to them – especially if we badger our doctors and let them know that we don't intend to suffer. And this applies just as much to women doctors as it does to the rest of womankind. I simply wouldn't tell everyone at work because, until the entire world is thoroughly enlightened on the topic of women's cyclical complaints, there are still those who think that women are on to a soft option and shouldn't be given jobs if they consider themselves to be ill for several days every month. And there is always the office tease, ready to come up with some puerile practical joke just at the very moment that you are least able to handle it. Keep such explanations for the home front, and you'll find you have made a wise decision.

Now let's have a look at how the premenstrual syndrome affects the housewife and mother, and what can be done to cope within the context of the home environment.

7

The Premenstrual Syndrome: At Home

Are you at home all day, and do you suffer from premenstrual syndrome symptoms every month? If so – and some of your friends who also have to contend with this complaint have a daily job to go to – you may find, to your surprise and indignation, that you are envied. This is because many people wrongly suppose that you have a far easier time than your employed friends who, regardless of how they feel, have to turn up for work.

You, they think, are in a position to take things gently when you do not feel well, and do not share their problems of rush-hour travel, difficult bosses and the demands of a regular nine-to-five job; nor the worry of your efficiency being impaired every month, possibly in a noticeable way. This way of thinking may be shared by your family, who feel that you have little cause for complaint and none whatever for snappiness or uneven temper because, unlike them, you don't have to cope with the daily stresses of life at the office, or at school or college.

What they forget, however, is that as a housewife and mother, you are tied to your place of work twenty-four hours a day, and cannot leave it behind you with a sigh of relief at five o'clock in the evening. You may well have your share of travel problems to face, if you take your husband to the station and/or the children to school. And who is to say that lowered efficiency in running a house and looking after small children affects you less than it affects your working friends in their employed capacities?

There are a number of advantages to having a paid job outside the home, however disinclined one feels when premenstrual to make the effort to go to it. The most obvious one is that, if you are at home because you cannot find a job, you lack the one morale-boosting fact that is of benefit to an employee, i.e. that someone, somewhere wants to employ your skills. There is also the financial problem of being out of work, and this is a considerable stress factor in the lives of many people, not least the premenstrual woman who monthly goes through a phase in which she is prone to depression and self-doubt in any case.

Besides the practical advantages of employment, having an outside job to go to imposes a form of discipline which can, in moderation, be of great help to the premenstrual sufferer. Certainly there are travel hazards and a number of predictable stresses during the day. But having to get up and go to work can sometimes act as a counter-stimulant to depression. If the depression is severe, no amount of external obligation or responsibility is likely to lift the heavy veil of inertia and lowered vitality. But a tendency to mild-to-moderate depressive illness can sometimes be successfully overcome by the obligation of effort and activity that a job involves. Even if the real stimulus is no more than the irritation of 'having to do something'.

Looking on the bright side, however, there are some very real benefits to being at home, and in this Chapter I will endeavour to outline them and point out how you can use them to the best advantage.

Discipline – by which I mean nothing harsher than a planned routine – forms the framework of any satisfactory day, and unless you are a DJ or work on Breakfast Television, yours is likely to conform to the common pattern of waking and getting up at a suitable time, and hopefully going to bed late enough to allow yourself a little evening recreation but not so late that you have insufficient sleep.

The worst thing you can do, if you suffer from the premenstrual syndrome and spend your days at home, is to let the day fall into pieces around you, or drag on wearily hour after hour without your achieving anything. A chosen routine should include the jobs you have to get done – for their own sake and yours so that you derive a sense of accomplishment out of performing them – and the pleasurable activities you hope to enjoy and which, if you like, you can regard as a reward for your efforts. If you ask cynically, 'What pleasurable activities?', when your day seems to consist of little besides small children, washing, ironing, cleaning and cooking, then your plan is not working as well as it might for you and it's time you rearranged things to suit you better.

Let's take the day at its earliest point, i.e. the moment at which you get out of bed. Not many people's favourite time, and considerably worse when you have a headache and sore breasts, and feel inert and tetchy. Whether you live alone, have a husband or lover who brings you tea in bed, or – more likely – have a lover or husband whom *you* wake with a drink, aim at getting out of bed on the 'right' side. The impressions that your senses receive and the path that your thoughts take in the first five minutes that you are awake after sleeping all night, invariably set the pattern for your mood, thoughts and feelings for the rest of the day. This is why you owe it to yourself to make your first impressions of the day favourable. The secret is to *allow yourself time*. Even if you are fully alert rather than semi-comatose on waking, do be kind to your body and mind and give them a few minutes to readjust to the conscious world. Your body has hopefully been relaxed and your mind free from inhibitions and control for a few blessed hours; it is just too much to expect them to click into motion and cope with mundane complexities the second your eyes are open and you realize that you are already ten minutes late!

Set your alarm twenty minutes early – it really isn't as ghastly an experience as all that – and allow yourself to 'come to' gradually. If you are habitually woken too early anyway, by the patter or thump of tiny or medium-sized feet, and the eager cries of: 'Mummy, Mummy' as the duvet on your side is pulled back, then muster your courage and exert the discipline over your child that you have a right to exert. Make him stay in his bedroom until *you* are ready to wake. This is not impossibly unrealistic. Basically all normal children, with effort on your part, can be trained to keep to certain rules. And if you allow some leeway, for instance, he can switch on his bedroom light and look at a book or play a game quietly until you are ready, you are likely to get co-operation in the end – even if you have to resort to the reward and punishment system to achieve it!

There you are then, lying there with twenty minutes to spare. You feel premenstrual; but try thinking some positive thoughts about the day ahead, and stretch luxuriously, yawning widely and gradually getting the muscles of your limbs to respond, before you sit up and get the day into motion. Whatever your usual morning routine, it is a good idea to make the time as relaxed as possible. Try laying the breakfast table the night before, even including such details as putting a spoonful of coffee or a teabag in each cup or mug and filling up the kettle and thawing or squeezing fresh fruit juice. Tidy up roughly before you go to bed, or get the last person up to do so, emptying ashtrays and waste-paper baskets, and throwing out crumpled newspapers. Most important, do not subject your early-morning self, particularly when premenstrual, to the depressing spectacle of last night's dinner or supper debris. If you give a dinner party, try nipping out between the courses to wash up as you go along – or accept sincere offers from any guests other than current or potential bosses to give you a hand. As a last stand, ask for a dishwasher for a combined birthday and Christmas present, pointing out what the outlay will contribute in terms of marital harmony. This machine can be worth its weight in gold encrusted platinum, if you're anxious to avoid rows first thing.

See also that the children, if you have them, have adequate selections of clothes and can find their school uniforms in the morning. You can only be certain of this if they get them out of the wardrobe, airing cupboard or wherever, before going to bed – another area for you to flex your disciplinary muscles, but they shouldn't really object when they discover the advantages to themselves. Also see that any packed lunches are prepared the evening or afternoon before – or make sandwiches a week in advance and keep them in the freezer or icebox, defrosting them as you need them.

Whatever means you plan to adopt, keep one principle in mind. Your object is to make life pleasant and relatively easy for yourself during your premenstrual phase – better still if you do so every morning. But we are concerned at the moment with avoiding a black mood when you wake, and the consequent descent of the day that can so easily happen, accompanied only too often by rows with loved ones and the risk of actual physical assault. Avoid the obviously sordid and stressful situations, and make your environment as aesthetic and calming, when you wake feeling tense and cross, as you would secretly like to see it. You will find your day gets off to a very much better start.

The less you are 'obliged' to do during the day, the more assiduously do you need to regulate your time to avoid falling into that limbo of almost-lost souls whose days lack any form of organization – and who consequently become demoralized, unproductive and totally unfulfilled. They become inefficient because they get out of the habit of planning their own lives, or cannot anyway as it has always been done for them. It is men and women such as these who eventually number among the unemployable, and occasionally turn to drink or drugs in order to derive some sort of a meaning from living.

If you have a lot to do during the day, then you will find that events to a certain extent take over and the natural sequence of your activities forms the skeleton of your timetable. Children are a great asset in preventing your days from running away from you. They have to be fed regularly, dressed in the morning if small and taken to school before they are old enough to go alone; they also come home needing food, drink and attention, usually simultaneously.

If you are feeling stressed, weepy and unattractive, it is only too easy to shelve visits to the shops, leave the housework and cancel bookings with your dentist, optician or hairdresser; so, if you have children of school age and do not go out to work, try the following plan for the premenstrual phase of your monthly cycle.

If you hate visiting the dentist at the best of times, then avoid making appointments to see him when you know your powers of endurance and physical stamina are at their lowest. On the other hand, deliberately book a session at your hairdresser's and, if you can afford it, have a facial and full make-up at the same time or, at the very least, a manicure. Any skilled attention to your body is money well spent; but the therapeutic effect on your morale and spirits of looking good is incalculable. It will be nice for the family to see you looking attractive and cheerful instead of drab and grumpy when they get in. But remember that your real reason for going to a beauty parlour or hair salon, is to benefit *you*.

The worst service you can do yourself (probably only practicable if you live alone anyway), is to surrender to bad early-morning miseries and stay in bed for the day. You may well find that the urge grows greater and greater, and eventually you may need what amounts almost to rehabilitation, before you are able to live successfully and productively again.

Try to organize your time along similar lines to those I have advised a busy office worker to follow. Look at your menstrual chart and note when your next premenstrual phase will be; make an effort to see that these days involve least stress for you. Arrange tiring jobs, such as taking all the curtains to the dry cleaners or stocking up your freezer, for other days of the month and try pampering yourself a little instead. And avoid starting a major task (such as a complete spring-clean, or wallpapering or painting a large room), during the week leading up to your premenstrual phase if it is too heavy a job for you to feel comfortable doing when affected by fluid retention and headaches, and you'd fret if it weren't finished.

If you happen to derive real pleasure from the creative side of this type of work, then by all means save all or part of such an undertaking for your premenstrual phase when you can really enjoy it and have very little time for succumbing to the 'blues', lethargy or inertia. But, unless you are built like an Amazon, still avoid really heavy labour which involves lifting or moving furniture or other cumbersome equipment. Congestive pelvic pain does not respond kindly to extra physical strain and could in fact be a great deal more troublesome if you approach hard work in the wrong way. If you have any tendency to develop asthma attacks, other allergic illness or migraines, it is a good idea to leave painting until you are well over the premenstrual syndrome, because of the recognized connection between the fumes produced by modern chemicals and the complaints I have mentioned. You have an increased proneness to all of these during your premenstrual phase, as we saw when we considered the physical symptoms of the illness.

Remember, too, before you climb step-ladders and perform impressive feats of daring at ceiling level, that you may become dizzy while doing so and that your powers of co-ordination may be a little impaired.

Other golden rules include: performing the same stretch and bend exercises that I recommended in the previous chapter, for the same reasons, and not missing breakfast! I do not have a fixation about the meal, and would do my best to correct a similar obsession in any patient who appeared to have one – but eating and drinking within the first hour of rising does make eminent sense if you aim to achieve something worthwhile during your sixteen or so hours of wakefulness.

Even if you do not eat with your husband, lover or children, wash up as soon as they have left the house and treat yourself to a cup of tea or coffee, preferably on the weak side, as it has been suggested that some women crave these beverages in extra strong concentration during their premenstrual phase because their systems get addicted to their caffeine content. And try a little home-made muesli with your drink – preferably one that is not too bulky and overfilling, and not too much trouble to make! The following is delicious and quickly made: put the juice of two oranges into a bowl and grate into this four eating apples. Add two tablespoonsful of sultanas, two rounded tablespoonsful each of milled cashew nuts and porridge oats and a little runny honey to taste. Eat some moistened with ordinary milk or top of the milk. This quantity is enough for two to three mornings, depending upon how much you like it!

If muesli is not your scene, treat yourself to a warm croissant, preferably wholemeal and yeasty, together with a little butter or Flora. And drink some freshly-squeezed juice beforehand. Whatever you choose you will be doing yourself a very good turn physically. Your metabolic system will be saved from the fate of having to launch itself into a day's activities without any fuel. It is like starting out on a day's drive in your car and refusing to refuel it so that it is obliged to manage as best it may on the remnants of yesterday's petrol. It would be silly to feel annoyed if you ran out of steam mid-morning and ground to a halt.

Along these lines, see that you have a snack every three hours or so while you are suffering from the premenstrual syndrome. I advised a premenstrual first-aid kit for office workers and others away from home all day; you do not really need this as everything you want is at your disposal when you are at home. But try to remember to eat something mid-morning and mid-afternoon, as well as having regular if small meals. This is to avoid attacks of hypoglycaemia (low blood sugar) to which you have a tendency when premenstrual, as the hormonal imbalance is associated with a lowering of your blood sugar from its normal level. There is no need to eat more than usual – in fact, avoid doing so if you already feel fat and bloated, because overeating (or to be blunt, absolutely stuffing and bingeing) makes you feel a whole lot worse. Just make certain that you do not go for too long without a snack or part-meal. If overeating due to intense food cravings is one of your premenstrual symptoms, stock up on non-fattening food items *which you enjoy*, and see that you get treatment for premenstrual illness as soon as possible. Overeating, and the consequent weight gain, followed by desperate measures to lose weight again before 'next time', is a frightening and destructive vicious circle in which to get caught up, both because real obesity is a serious health hazard and because feeling unattractive, when there is a remedy at hand, is unnecessarily and sadly soul-destroying.

I often recommend the following routine to women 'stuck at home' and suffering from the premenstrual syndrome, when they ask for specific advice on *how* to reorganize themselves when they are depressed, inert and frankly bored. Leave yourself minimal serious household chores and after breakfast while still in your dressing gown or housecoat, finish the tidying, and flit around with duster and carpet-sweeper. Save hoovering for a non-premenstrual day, or for whichever household member dares to criticize you for being sufficiently lazy to use the carpet-sweeper! Seriously, if you can inveigle a son or daughter into hoovering the night before, so much the better. You should ask your husband – but either he already does it for you on difficult days, or he'd die of shock at being asked! Do a few other obvious things, such as throwing out dead flowers, squaring up the bathroom after the early morning's onslaught upon its usual pristine neatness and re-laying and lighting the fire, if it is winter time or winter-minded weather and you are fortunate enough to have a coal fire.

Then run yourself a bath, add some delicious-smelling oil or bubbles and soak. Play the radio or a cassette while you're there and have a thoroughly hedonistic three-quarters of an hour, followed by a hair-wash and dry, the application of fresh nail varnish and some attractive make-up. Then, back in the bedroom, devote a couple of minutes to stretching and bending, if you didn't have time before breakfast. The final step in your morning preparations – and very important it is – is the choice of what to wear. If you normally do not bother, because there's no one there to see, just remember that *you* are the most important person in your life today, and *you* care how you look because it is essential that you feel good. You have more freedom of choice than someone who works for a boss – so exercise it! If your stomach isn't particularly swollen, opt for your favourite pair of jeans – preferably the stretch variety – and a good bra and a warm (or cool), pretty top. If you are or feel enormous and bloated, go for a loose-cut dress in a soft, flattering colour, or a track suit or a non-constricting jumpsuit.

The message is – look and feel as good as you can. There is another reason for this. Many women experience profound feelings of inadequacy, ugliness and unworthiness when the psychological manifestations of the premenstrual syndrome affect them severely. This is often an aspect of the depression so common then, or may be part of a temporary inclination to 'hide away' until it is all over because morale, together with sex drive and self-confidence, is at an all-time low. At home all day, many women seek some sort of reassurance, albeit unconsciously, and check in the mirror time and again to make certain that they don't look that offensive/disgusting/repulsive. If their mirror image is wearing make-up, nice clothes and fresh nail varnish, and has clean, shiny hair and a reasonably cheerful expression, the effect will be restorative rather than destructive. When the reverse is true, and they find they look worse than even they had imagined possible, the effect is quite the opposite.

You are now in a position to face the day with a certain amount of self-confidence. Try to make sure that this is not impaired by attempting and failing to rush through too many jobs, by the behaviour of your children, the next-door neighbour, erratic postal deliveries, unexpected telephone calls or the sudden arrival of one or several dinner guests whom your husband forgot to mention to you. There are some things we just can't control, so try not to be thrown by them.

I've stated that your day ought to be constructive, and pointed out the types of jobs that are unsuitable for you to tackle at that time. But you should give yourself a definite objective to achieve each day, nevertheless – and the premenstrual phase affords an excellent opportunity to start and complete a sewing job; write some letters – business and personal; tidy out a cupboard or two; and do some baking for your freezer. If you do not own a freezer, then you can treat yourself to far less cooking the next week, by having a baking session and making cakes, pies, tarts (filled and unfilled), biscuits and bread, thereby impressing your family with your industry as well as pleasantly delighting their taste-buds – once you have become a competent baker!

If this sort of cooking is new to you, buy or borrow a reliable book on the subject and try out some of the recipes with the aid of a friend. Bread baking is, in fact, very therapeutic, for not only are you dealing with earthy, satisfying, basic ingredients such as flour, salt and yeast, which placate the soul, but the more you knead bread dough (within reason!) the better it rises when cooked – and kneading is an excellent way of working off accumulated frustrations. I can never see the point of breaking tons of crockery. Unless you go out into the park with a complete dinner service (just think of carrying that half a mile, in a suitcase!) you only have the irritating task of clearing all the mess up afterwards as a sort of symbolic punishment for having lost control. Far better to slap, punch and belt the life out of a piece of harmless dough, then fling it into a prepared tin, get it into a pre-set oven, and enjoy the delightful smells that come issuing forth after ten minutes or so as you wash down the work surface. Best of all is its flavour, when you break off a piece while it is still hot and eat it buttered and redolent of yeast.

Whatever you choose to do in the way of chores when premenstrual – see that you don't get too tired and see that you enjoy it.

What if you are a freelance worker, and carry on your occupation at home? Do make the effort to bath, dress attractively, keep your home pleasant to be in, and frustration to a minimum. But as you fit in between the externally-employed worker and the housewife engaged in running a home full-time, you will probably want to leave visits to the hairdresser and other such pursuits to the weekend. It is very difficult to exert constant self-discipline such as is needed to work effectively at home. So it is essential that you think up a plan that will work with respect to your division of available time – and stick to it.

At least when you are your own boss, you can get up and go out for a walk when you get thoroughly fed up with the typewriter, knitting machine, easel and palette or tape-recorder. Just make certain that you are a little easier on yourself on premenstrual days, but at the same time try to keep to your usual routine. Probably the most stressful home-based occupation you can be involved in, especially when irritable, headachey and exhausted, is looking after babies or small children. They are, of course, at the same time a great source of joy and happiness, and very few mothers indeed would elect to be free from the responsibility of rearing their children, but not one of the euphemisms pertaining to the bliss of motherhood compensates, at the time, for mopping up vomit, rinsing out soiled underpants and nappies, and feeling so tired that you are convinced you'll simply keel over and die.

Everyone who has read books on child rearing knows that our children 'respond to our moods'. That's fine – all the time we are in a happy state of mind. But it is equally true that whenever one feels irritable, lethargic and definitely too frail to cope with fractious infants – that is the one time babies and toddlers can be relied upon to play up. The worse your headache, the harder you strive to control your temper – it isn't their fault, you reason, why should they suffer just because you are premenstrual and feel absolutely grotty? Very true, but if you have to control your urge to hit them too often and too hard, then the danger signs are there for you to take notice of. Many children do get injured, not necessarily by a drunken father or a fighting mother, but at times by a parent (in this case let's say a premenstrual mum), who suddenly snaps, and hits out before she is able to control herself. If you think this could apply to you, please do something about it now, before the deed is done. I am not only thinking about the very real danger to your child; I am equally concerned about the damage injuring your child does to you, both in terms of acute remorse and resultant self-hatred, and very possibly to your marital or stable love relationship.

By all means have treatment for the premenstrual syndrome as outlined in this book. It will very likely work wonders for the way you feel, and in a month or two you will be and feel a very different person. But in the meantime, see your doctor if he or she is an understanding kind of person, and/or have a word with a friend or neighbour about your worries. Talking about fears can do a lot to allay them and this is a problem in which you are not alone. If you are desperate for someone to talk to and cannot confide in a friend, try the Samaritans who are, perhaps, the world's very best listeners.

There is another thing that you can do to tide you over this dangerous period: discuss the matter with your husband or lover, speaking frankly about your fears – providing the relationship will stand up to this revelation. It could be of benefit, in that it may indicate just how badly you need understanding help and treatment. Then arrange for someone you can trust (relative, friend, baby-minder, day nursery) to have your young children for an hour or so each day, and for longer when your premenstrual phase comes up.

Finally, to help yourself in this parlous situation and to cope better throughout the premenstrual syndrome generally, arrange to have adequate exercise. Take a walk to the park every day; and if you work at home, try to get the equivalent of an office girl's share of exertion and take a walk in the morning and the evening. Try taking your lunch out to eat in a local quiet square or on a park bench – and if you are engaged full time in running the house, try lunch in the park and a trip to the shops when they are least likely to be busy. You may very well feel that it is not worth the effort when you are feeling low, dispirited and fatigued, but the fresh air will help you to think more clearly and to concentrate better, just as the walk will improve your circulation, tone up your muscles, give you a better complexion and whip some colour into your cheeks. It will also fight off the deep cloud of despondency you may well be labouring under, and give you a sense of having achieved something. Besides walking, there are many other forms of exercise that could suit you at this time, depending on how the premenstrual syndrome affects you. If your bugbear is a feeling of nerviness and tension, swimming several lengths of a swimming pool could restore a sense of well-being and relaxation; so could a round of squash or a couple of games of table tennis. If you have the greatest reluctance to drag one foot after another, opt for a brisk ten-minute walk instead!

The whole point is to strike a suitable balance between conforming to a routine and recreation, between having adequate rest and sufficient exercise. Ask your family to help you in this respect and make them see that you need their help and co-operation. Every one of you should benefit from it.

8
The Premenstrual Syndrome: At School

If your periods started only recently, or if you are well into your teens and have been having periods for some time, have you considered whether you may suffer from the premenstrual syndrome too? The illness I have been discussing in the earlier chapters of this book more often affects women in their twenties or over. Generally speaking, painful periods are commoner in young girls and women and tend to get better as the years go by – especially after they have had a baby. This contrasts with premenstrual syndrome symptoms, which are rather more likely to get worse with the passage of time and sometimes make their first appearance *after* the birth of a baby.

These statements, however, are generalizations, and while they are true of a large majority of women, they tell us nothing about the individual person. It is just as possible to suffer from the premenstrual syndrome in the early years of your reproductive life, as it is to suffer from severe spasmodic dysmenorrhoea (painful periods), right up to the time when your periods stop at the menopause.

We've distinguished between painful periods as such and the group of symptoms that together constitute the premenstrual syndrome. They are different from one another and therefore require different kinds of treatment. As I pointed out earlier, you would be very unlucky indeed – and unlikely – to suffer from both complaints; but do not make the mistake of thinking that because you are young you could not be suffering from premenstrual illness since this belongs to an older age group. Many girls and women are very tense and irritable while they are waiting for their periods to begin, and it was due to the fact that tension is such a prominent feature of premenstrual illness that the old name 'premenstrual tension' became popular. But, as we have seen, this is an inaccurate way of describing the condition which in reality consists of a complex mixture of physical and mental symptoms.

If you have read the two chapters dealing with these symptoms, you may now be able to attribute some of your own experiences to a hormonal imbalance – experiences which perhaps have puzzled or alarmed you as you did not know their cause. These could have included painful breasts, frequent headaches and acne which have recurred for no apparent reason from time to time, and the best way to discover whether these are premenstrual symptoms is to fill in the menstrual chart detailed in Chapter 6. If necessary, you can fill in the symptom score chart as well.

Another problem the chapter on psychological symptoms may solve is why at certain times in the month you are far more likely to row with your parents, other members of your family, your boyfriend and/or your closest girlfriend. And why, round about these times, you may feel shy, unsure of yourself and unwilling to go out, whereas normally you adore going to discos, the pub or out to enjoy a favourite sport.

This can be worrying and distressing if you are not aware of the cause. It is harder for you in many respects, than it is for women of other age groups with the premenstrual syndrome, to appreciate that shortness of temper, irritability and tearfulness could be caused by changes taking place in your glands every month due to a deficiency of fatty acids. For it is very usual for girls of your age group to experience emotional difficulties and feel out of sorts with society generally, as well as angry and frustrated at the poor communication between older people and teenagers. You probably row with your parents from time to time anyway, because they try to impose rules on you that your friends are not expected to obey –

or because you feel that they are old-fashioned, narrow, restrictive and incapable of understanding you.

It is perfectly 'normal', although somewhat hard on both you and your parents and other adults, when you feel and act rebelliously, and, premenstrual syndrome aside, this interaction can reasonably be expected to form a part of every teenager's developing years. It is emotionally traumatic for all concerned, especially for you – but does not necessarily mean that you are suffering from premenstrual illness. If, on the other hand, filling in the symptoms on your two charts reveals that you are consistently far more irritable, tense and weepy in the days leading up to your period, you should suspect that this may be the cause.

Evidence of the premenstrual miseries on your chart will more than likely be supported by other suggestive facts such as the regular occurrence during this time of acne and spots (or a worsening in your usual skin trouble), sore, tender breasts and – perhaps the hardest thing to put up with – a weight increase. Suspect the premenstrual syndrome as the likely culprit and discuss the problem with your mother after she has read this book. If either of you is in any doubt that this is the cause of your trouble, go and have a chat with your doctor, with or without your mother, depending on how you normally approach these things. Do not forget, though, to take your chart or charts along with you to show the doctor. At least two months' symptoms should have been filled in to demonstrate the regular appearance of your complaints in the days leading up to your monthly periods.

Here's what to do once you, and anybody else you have discussed the matter with, are convinced that you are affected by the premenstrual syndrome. Take a look at the list of physical symptoms first, to work out how you can best cope with them within the context of a busy school day.

Tender breasts
If this is your problem, wear a looser bra and put out of your mind the fear that you have got some dreadful disease, however painful and swollen they might be. But if you can feel anything like a lump or hard area, go along to see your doctor, who will examine you and doubtless reassure you that you have nothing to worry about.

Some teenage girls find this idea very embarrassing, particularly if their breasts are either just starting to develop or are larger than is currently fashionable. If you don't like the idea of a male doctor touching your breasts, try to make an appointment with the lady doctor partner. There is one in most group practices nowadays and many women of all ages prefer to talk to another woman about female problems. If this is not possible – because the lady doctor is non-existent, away on holiday or too booked up – don't put up with your worry in secret for weeks on end. Ask your mother, sister or school friend to accompany you; the examination does not take many seconds and do remember that any GP, in the course of a week in practice, sees the rectums, vaginas, penises, fat stomachs and ugly feet of many dozens of old, young, skinny, overweight, attractive, plain, pleasant and thoroughly cantankerous people – and quite honestly, examining breasts is no more exciting or remarkable to him or her than taking the wrappings off plaster models is to a window-dresser. So relax and do go if you are worried. At least it will set your mind at rest.

Weight gain

During the premenstrual phase of a woman's monthly cycle, her weight can increase by anything from a couple of pounds to a stone. If your weight is affected in this way, do at least comfort yourself with the fact that the dilemma is due to the retention of fluid which will be lost again quite quickly once your period has started. It is not caused by some cruel and callous fate which decrees that you will never achieve your target weight, regardless of how much you diet and exercise. For this reason, do not allow the scales to upset you, and do not try to rectify matters by going on a drastic diet at that very time of the month when you are prone to attacks of low blood sugar anyway. If you use the menstrual chart properly, you will see that there is a corresponding fall in the amount of urine that you pass in a day during this time. And this can make you quite certain that your weight gain is caused by the factors I have discussed.

Try to eat normally, neither starving nor bingeing. This takes us conveniently to the next physical symptom.

Abnormal food cravings

I call them 'abnormal' because most of us at some time experience a sudden strong desire for a particular item to eat or drink. Pregnant women are generally supposed to have the monopoly of *abnormal* cravings of this type, and their unexpected and intense need for fresh pineapple chunks, prawn dhansak or condensed milk at the least convenient times has long been attributed to hormonal changes.

As we have seen, changes in hormonal pattern, due to the lack of fatty acids, plays a prominent part in premenstrual illness, and these, too, are capable of causing cravings for food items that are so irresistible that diets and 'good' eating habits are abandoned. The girl or woman, normally a strict dieter or at least someone who is very careful about her calorie intake, suddenly binges on outrageously rich and fattening junk foods and adds several pounds of actual fat to her transitory weight problem of extra fluid.

If you are tormented by a longing for spoonfuls of sugar in your drinks, cream-filled chocolates or jam doughnuts by the dozen, this is very likely due either to emotional stress, depression or tension (which will be discussed later), or to the physical fact of your blood-sugar level falling as a result of hormone imbalance. The best way to counteract this is to see that you do not go for longer than three hours without a snack. Whether you eat school meals or take a packed lunch with you, do remember to take something extra to eat during the morning break and make certain that you eat before leaving home in the morning. A piece of toast or bowl of cereal may be all that you can manage, but if you keep to the rule of eating just a little before starting your day, again at break, at lunch-time and soon after getting out of school, you are unlikely to suffer from acute hunger pangs and severe cravings, and thus ruin your diet.

Swelling (stomach, fingers, wrists and ankles)
Because your body is retaining much more fluid than usual, rather than getting rid of it by means of the urine that you pass, parts of you get correspondingly fatter, for the extra fluid has to be stored *somewhere*. The parts most likely to be affected are your stomach (abdomen), fingers, wrists and ankles, and you will notice that the waistbands of skirts and trousers feel tight and uncomfortable. Rings and watch-straps may be difficult to get on, and your calf muscles and feet may ache.

Avoid putting any extra salt on your food for a couple of days before that point in your cycle when you expect premenstrual symptoms to commence, and avoid salty snacks such as nuts, crisps, etc. You could leave your rings off for a day or two while you are waiting for the swelling to subside, and try carrying your watch round with you in a safe pocket. And if your waist does expand uncomfortably every month, add an extra hook or button on your skirt waistband so that you can let it out without any fuss when you need to do so. This is a bit of a nuisance job – but well worth the effort compared to feeling unbearably constricted around the middle for several days every month where your normal waistband pinches you.

Muscular aches and pains
You may well be familiar with period pains, which affect most women who suffer from them as a deep-down, dragging sensation in the pelvic region, accompanied either by stomach-ache or by low backache. Pain can be felt, too, in the upper parts of the thighs and in the outer genital region and the deep, nagging ache can make you feel very unwell and disinclined to activity.

Period pain is called spasmodic dysmenorrhoea because it is produced by certain muscles going into a cramp-like spasm as the blood and lining of your womb is pushed out to the exterior. But as I explained in Chapter 3, the pain or dysmenorrhoea of the premenstrual phase is due to the congestion and swelling of blood vessels in the organs of your pelvis.

What should you do when you are suffering from severe pelvic discomfort and face a hectic day ahead at school? Before I discuss the treatment of the complete premenstrual syndrome in detail, I will just mention the subject of pain-killers. If you do decide to take any, go for the milder ones such as aspirin or paracetamol, and buy the soluble rather than the insoluble type. They are not too bad to taste when dissolved in a glass of water, especially if you add a squeeze of fresh lemon or orange juice to the glass, and they are absorbed more rapidly than the solid tablets you swallow whole. This means that they enter the bloodstream more rapidly, and can get to work to relieve your pain at the earliest possible opportunity. Do not take them on an empty stomach, though. Have at least a glass of milk or a couple of biscuits first, and avoid aspirin if you suffer from any sort of gastric trouble, or if you've had stomach pain in the past as a result of taking them.

The secret of obtaining relief from pain with mild pain-killers is to take them at the earliest indication that you are going to need them. Don't just take them to school with you, hoping for an opportunity to slip into the cloakroom, find a convenient glass of water, and swallow them down at break. As soon as you feel a twinge that you are certain is going to develop into considerable discomfort, find your pills and take them at once – preferably before leaving home in the morning.

The other variety of pain for which this treatment might be useful is that which affects your joints and the muscles of your limbs, neck and back. It is thought to be due to the fact that you are extra tense at this time and tend to hold yourself stiffly. If you are interested in yoga, and either go to classes in your spare time or attend a course at school, do go on with them. Yoga teaches muscular control, excellent posture and relaxation, and all of these can help you a great deal to overcome your premenstrual discomfort.

With respect to swimming, games and gym, if you are a sports enthusiast and the pain is not too severe, go ahead and join in. You will probably find that a session on the netball court or hockey pitch will work wonders for your pent-up energy and tension, and that your pain will be far less troublesome. On the other hand, if your pain is bad and has not responded to the pain-killers you have taken earlier, have a word with the sports mistress or deputy headmistress, or get your mother to write a note on your behalf excusing you from strenuous activity.

Physical clumsiness
The movements of a minority of people are graceful and deft at all times. Those of many of us tend to be clumsy and heavy-handed. If you belong to the latter type, you may well find that you are teased about the frequency with which you drop and break things, and the way you are involved in minor accidents generally. This can be very annoying, particularly during your premenstrual phase when many women are more prone to physical clumsiness than at any other time. If this is a major problem for you, because you hate being teased and laughed at, try relaxation methods from a good

book on the subject, or yoga. Try also to be less uptight about the matter as inner tension only makes things worse. If you practise the art, you will be able to take people's teasing in good part. They probably don't mean any harm and a good remedy is sometimes to find one of their oddities to tease them about in return.

Where you must take poor physical co-ordination seriously, is when you are faced with a gym lesson in which you usually partake of spectacular manoeuvres at the top of ropes and on vaulting horses. If you have a pronounced tendency to fall, trip or stumble during your premenstrual phase, do avoid performing activities of this type and, whatever you do, do it close to ground level! You may have an excellent head for heights when performing gymnastics under normal conditions, but spells of nausea and dizziness affect many women premenstrually and can come on quite unexpectedly. This is another reason for avoiding dangerous activities if you are affected by premenstrual symptoms.

Skin disorders

Acne, spots, pimples and other types of skin blemishes are extremely common during the teenage years. This is in part due to the hormonal changes which you are going through in your development to full maturity. Many girls and women are especially prone to bad skin during the premenstrual phase of their cycle – but simply knowing the reason why your skin is in a bad condition is not much of a compensation when you had hoped to look radiantly attractive for a special party you are going to, or out on a date with a new boyfriend.

The usual advice for teenage acne is equally applicable to the skin disorders caused by premenstrual illness, and includes the use of a mildly-medicated soap, and the avoidance of too many fatty foods, particularly chocolate, chips and other fried foods. Start to take extra care of your skin a day or two before you expect it to grow worse – which fact you will be able to tell from looking at your premenstrual chart. Be stricter than usual about what you eat and drink and try at the same time to include several glasses of tap or bottled water in your daily fluid intake. Eat as much salad, vegetables and fruit as you can manage and take at least some outdoor exercise daily.

Your school may or may not allow you to use make-up, but

there is no reason why you should not disguise bad spots by means of masker cream which is available in pencil or stick form, or in a small bowl container. At night, wash off the cream, dry your skin carefully and apply a little antiseptic ointment on red or sore areas.

If acne remains a problem, see your doctor who will probably prescribe one of the several types of acne treatment made by pharmaceutical companies. The treatment for the premenstrual syndrome that I shall be discussing in the next two chapters, however, is often remarkably effective in improving the condition of the skin.

Eczema, which is in many instances an allergic reaction, can be worse than usual during the premenstrual syndrome too; and this responds very well indeed to the new therapy.

Allergic conditions

If you tend to be allergic to a wide variety of substances from strawberries to penicillin, you will probably find that this tendency is enhanced during the days immediately before your period starts. This can be very aggravating because, in addition to your less-than-perfect skin condition of acne and blemishes, the last thing you want is a collection of red blotches, swelling and rashes.

If, too, you are unfortunate enough to suffer from asthma, you may discover that you get more attacks during the premenstrual phase. These are two very valid reasons for being treated for the basic underlying cause of the premenstrual syndrome so that all these tendencies are counteracted at source.

Migraine attacks

Besides allergic conditions, you may suffer from an increased sensitivity to certain foods, such as cheese, oranges and chocolate, resulting in migraine attacks. There is a recognized association between migraine and these food items anyway, and you may find that you get the occasional migraine attack at other times as well, but are much more likely to succumb during the days leading up to your period.

The best answer is to try correcting the premenstrual syndrome first, and in the meantime equip yourself with a reliable brand of anti-migraine remedy, either by buying them from your chemist (eg. Migraleve in the duo-pack form) or asking your doctor to prescribe something for you. Take whatever you settle on according to the directions, and at the earliest possible sign that an attack may be about to start. Also avoid any foodstuffs which you have found tend to induce an attack in you – these include the ones I have mentioned, and alcohol as well!

Don't attempt to go to school if you have a real migraine underway or threatening to start. You can tell whether your head pains constitute migraine attacks or are non-migrainous severe headaches, in the following way. Migraine sufferers generally notice various visual disturbances which herald an attack, such as partial blindness, flashing, coloured lights and shooting stars. The headache, too, is usually typical and at first involves one side of the head only – in which position it may stay, or from which it may radiate to involve the entire head. Affected people nearly always go very pale, and nausea and vomiting are a prominent feature in many cases. Their eyes become painfully sensitive to light, which they cannot bear, and in a severe attack they can only lie still in a quiet, darkened room until therapy takes effect or the attack naturally subsides.

Now that we've seen the range of problems that the physical symptoms of the premenstrual syndrome can present when you are at school, we will take a look at the emotional side of this illness and work out how best to cope with it.

Tension

The sensation of inner tension is always an excessively unpleasant one, and in Chapters 7 and 8 I reviewed the ways in which this symptom can affect the older woman: first, when she is at work all day, and then when she spends the day at home as a housewife, as a mother of small children, and/or as a freelance worker working from home.

The physical symptoms I mentioned as accompanying tension, such as a rapid heartbeat, shortness of breath, etc., naturally apply just as much to you, a teenager at school; but I want to focus upon the manner of coping best with intensely frustrated feelings, both in the classroom and when you get home.

There is no moral side to this advice. My whole object is to suggest how best to manage, by giving yourself the least stress. By trial and error, I have eventually found this advice to be the most successful – just don't fight anybody! Try to be slow to react to what you may think of as deliberate attempts to irritate you, by refusing to get irritated – either by your parents, or your teachers, or your friends.

Make life as easy and simple for yourself as you possibly can – and this means doing a certain number of jobs at home, and as much homework as you can persuade yourself to do, simply because it is more trouble in the end *for you* if you do not, as you will then have to argue about it with someone. If you find yourself bursting into tears easily, and getting worked up about what is really very little provocation, don't add to your woes by feeling embarrassed and ashamed. It is safe to say that every single healthy girl or woman you meet, without exception, will have experienced some degree of emotional difficulty in her life in association with menstruation – either during her period, or before it (premenstrual tension). We all know what it is like to feel unbearably tense at such times, so don't feel worse – because you are afraid you have made a fool of yourself – or apologize profusely afterwards, unless you have been really insulting or deeply hurtful. Such things happen to the best *and* the worst of us, and it is nothing to get too worked up about.

Lack of sex drive
Whether you have a steady boyfriend with whom you make love regularly, or go out occasionally in groups and as yet have had no true sexual experience, recognizing the fact that your natural libido (sex drive) may be at an all-time low if you are affected by the premenstrual syndrome, can help you to cope when a boy makes a pass at you and you find it off-putting.

If he is your regular partner, don't let his feelings be hurt, and don't start worrying that you are frigid! Ask him whether he has heard of premenstrual symptoms, point out that you are one of the people affected by them – and ask him to be extra-specially understanding and loving to you. Explained in this way, the symptoms should make perfect sense to him – and if they don't and he gets upset, show him relevant parts of this book! If he is a new date, and you are not sure of him or how understanding he is likely to be, decide quickly whether he is worth explaining the situation to, or whether there seems to be little point in going into details about female complaints because he is not sufficiently mature to understand – or you are not sufficiently concerned to bother!

Not feeling like sex, or even a close embrace because your breasts are exceptionally tender, is *perfectly normal!* You do not have to apologize because you are affected in this way: most women are to a greater or lesser extent. You'll feel quite different once your period has started – and on top of the world, once it is over!

So don't worry, and don't let anyone you love worry, either.

Depression

This is a horrid symptom, and you may already be familiar with it as it occurs to a considerable extent during the teen years anyway, quite apart from the premenstrual syndrome. As well as feeling miserable, inadequate and antisocial, you may well feel strongly disinclined to participate in any group activities, preferring to keep yourself to yourself.

My advice is – don't force yourself. If you really want to be alone, seek every opportunity to achieve this loneness and do your own thing, whether it be listening to the Stones, reading T. S. Eliot's poems – or simply sleeping or daydreaming. The only time you ought to try to fight the solitary state is when you feel cross and awkward and drive everybody away, while secretly you long for a friendly and sympathetic listener. Under those circumstances, tell your mother, best friend or boyfriend how you feel and depend on their sympathy and loyalty. Who knows, your mother and best friend may very well be similarly affected and be trying to pluck up courage to tell you their troubles. Most girls and women can find reciprocal ways of helping one another if they put their minds to it!

If you get seriously depressed and fantasize about frankly morbid things such as death, suicide, or worse – do confide in somebody. The best person is your mother. The next best person is your dad, sister or brother or best friend. Otherwise trust a teacher, minister or your doctor if you know him. Whatever you do, don't put up with feeling utterly wretched for several days every month just because you cannot face telling anybody how you feel.

Treating the premenstrual syndrome may be all the therapy you need. If your depression is independent of this hormonal flux, then you require treatment and the sooner you have it, the better.

Lethargy and poor concentration

These symptoms are absolute bugbears when you are trying to do well at school or when you are about to revise/sit for an examination. See that you get plenty of sleep and enough outdoor exercise during the day to make good sleep more or less a certainty at night. If you can get some homework, or a home project, off the ground before your premenstrual symptoms start, this should help a very great deal.

Otherwise, go as gently with yourself as you can and try to see that neither you nor anyone else expects too much of you when you are premenstrual.

9

Alleviating the Symptoms

We saw earlier that, although 'premenstrual tension' had been recognized for three centuries and represented by a brief footnote in a number of medical textbooks since the seventeenth century, no one really paid much attention to it. Doctors and research workers did not become interested in it until the 'sixties and 'seventies, when women themselves started to complain and be more open about their monthly symptoms.

Called premenstrual tension for a long time, the illness became recognized as an entity which has been renamed the premenstrual syndrome since it was realized that there existed a whole complex of related physical and psychological symptoms of which tension and irritability are only the prominent tip of an iceberg.

But once names have captured the popular imagination they are slow to change, and the illness was still represented as 'PMT' (premenstrual tension) when it became headline news in the criminal cases I mentioned earlier. Since living in our society becomes increasingly stressful – and encountering a myriad of stressful stimuli during the premenstrual phase worsens the symptoms of this complaint – we have become increasingly aware of premenstrual syndrome in the Western hemisphere and much research has been conducted into its possible causes.

Fortunately for all of us in many ways, the medical profession and the pharmaceutical companies do not wait until the actual causes of an illness is brought to light before treating it. This may be a policy of perfection, but would do nothing whatever for the countless patients who suffered without treatment for their symptoms while the underlying bodily malfunction was being investigated. Symptomatic treatment is clearly second-best, for the discovery of the cause of an illness often suggests ways of treating the faulty mechanism responsible for it – and maybe eradicating the disease altogether. But sometimes treating symptoms is the only approach by which relief can be offered to patients.

Since the early 1970s, the premenstrual syndrome has fitted this category of 'symptomatic therapy only', while systematic investigations have been carried out into the 'whys and wherefores' of the complaint. Numerous types of treatment have been adopted, and most of them have afforded many women some relief. It was recognized, quite early on, that the swelling and weight gain of premenstrual women was due to the body retaining fluid instead of excreting it; and because of the hormonal changes that are known to take place during the premenstrual phase, premenstrual symptoms were quite naturally attributed to the actual hormonal imbalances that often arise then.

It is known that the excretion of fluid from the body, for example, or indeed its retention, is under the direct control of a hormone produced by the pituitary gland. And having settled on 'hormonal imbalance' as the explanation for premenstrual illness, few people looked further. Treatments were designed to combat and correct the hormonal 'highs' and 'lows', and the production of female hormones was exhaustively observed, tested and discussed.

The fact that this is not the whole story, and that the underlying problem is a deficiency within the body of essential fatty acids (EFAs), has only recently come to light. We will look in detail at the relationship between this deficiency and hormone imbalance shortly, but I must point out that although it is now believed that the cause has been isolated, nobody would be stupid enough to claim that the problem is not also largely hormonal. The discovery of the effects of a lack of EFAs complements and does not contradict many of the points of the hormonal theory. It is simply that hormonal abnormalities, and the way that the body reacts to them, is the result of its lack of EFAs, rather than the prime cause.

All the symptomatic treatment mentioned here is effective in a number of women. It does at best quell symptoms, but before the new treatment was available it was all that could be offered. It is worth trying if your problem is severe and you wish to help yourself as much as possible.

Fluid and salt restriction
It is obvious that if your kidneys are helping to retain fluid in your body rather than making urine in order to get rid of it, a good way to hinder this fluid retention is to cut down on the quantity of fluid that you drink. Take care not to go overboard about restricting your fluids, however, because water – in whatever form we take it – is essential to health and life.

Water accounts for fifty per cent of a woman's body weight (and sixty per cent of a man's body weight, the difference being due to the fact that on average women carry more fat than men, and fat contains no water). We inevitably lose about one and a half litres of water daily for the kidneys have to form at least 600 milli-litres (ml) of urine daily in order to get rid of toxic waste matter. Evaporation from the skin accounts for another 500 ml, and evaporation from the lungs, 300 ml. About 100 ml is lost in normal stools (a great deal more when diarrhoea is present).

All food contains some water, so eating replaces some of that which is lost. An average diet may provide 600 ml of 'free' water and in addition, we manufacture about 300 ml as the end-product of combustion, along with carbon dioxide. This means that the remaining 600 ml (about one pint) has to be replaced by drinking. This is the very least that must be drunk each day in cool surroundings, and remember that sweating can greatly increase the loss. In extreme conditions, the sweat glands are able to pour out as much as ten litres in one day!

You can help yourself by cutting down on the amount of salt you take. This means declining the offer of salt during mealtimes, avoiding obviously salty foods and possibly cooking without salt. Food, especially vegetables and bread, taste very odd prepared without this condiment, but if you persevere you can get used to

the difference, and start to notice that many foods have interesting
and subtle flavour undertones which were not discernible when
the flavour of salt predominated. There are also salt substitutes
that you can buy. These are available from health-food shops,
which started to sell them when it became known that one of the
reasons for elevated blood pressure in the West is the relatively
huge amount of salt that we consume every year.

Yoga and relaxation

Learning and practising yoga can help you in three ways, if you
suffer from the premenstrual syndrome. Firstly, the postures and
the breathing techniques are designed to instil a peaceful and
tranquil state in the practitioner – physically and mentally. We
have seen that the physical aspects of tension, such as tightness of
the muscles, painful joints, shallow and inefficient breathing and a
rapid heartbeat can be almost as troublesome as the mental aspects
of great inner turmoil and outbursts of irritability. Learning how
to control your breathing – in particular how to breathe slowly
and deeply – can eradicate both types of symptoms. The lessening
of tension in your muscles should help a lot, if muscular and joint
aches and pains trouble you.

The second way in which yoga helps many women is in
teaching the maintenance of an upright and balanced posture. This
is not difficult to learn if you persist, and it relieves much of the
fatigue and lethargy, as well as the low back pain, of many
premenstrual syndrome sufferers.

Thirdly, there are a number of yoga postures which are of
particular benefit to sufferers from congestive dysmenorrhoea.
They are the following: the Plough, the Fish, the Cobra,
Uddiyana and the Shoulder Stand. Figure 4 shows you what these
postures look like, but it is best to learn them from an experienced
teacher as you should start with an understanding of the basic
yogic principles and the easiest of the postures, before attempting
the advanced ones.

If yoga does not appeal to you, try attending relaxation classes.
You will find notices about classes and groups in the local
newspaper and on cards in high-street shop-windows and
tobacconists' display boards; your local library is also a likely place
to find out about courses, and you may get to hear of a group from

an interested neighbour or friend. The benefits of learning true relaxation are sometimes a revelation and a number of women who have been to such classes state that they had not relaxed in that way – ever before!

If you would prefer to follow any such pursuit in the privacy of your own home, go for relaxation tapes. This is a pleasant way to learn to relax and the advantage of it is that you can switch on the cassette or record whenever you feel inclined, and are not tied to attending lessons at a particular time each week. Classes can be fun, though, and are a good way of meeting people of similar interests and maybe with similar problems. If you opt for the 'home' method, remember to dim the lighting in the room you are using, take the telephone off its hook, and ignore the front-door bell. Also choose a time of day when you are not likely to be disturbed – cries of: 'Mummy, Mummy, come and look!' are not conducive to relaxation at its most beneficial!

Vitamin therapy

I have said sufficient on the topic of pyridoxine (vitamin B_6) in the treatment of the premenstrual syndrome for it to be quite clear that it can be very useful in some cases of this illness. Supplementary vitamin B_6 helps where the woman's requirement for it far exceeds the normal, as a result of hormone imbalance.

The particular symptoms that pyridoxine can help to relieve include premenstrual headache and depression, and it has special value for premenstrual women suffering from fluid retention. A pioneer in the clinical studies of this vitamin, John M. Ellis, MD, of Mount Pleasant, Texas, reports considerable success in the treatment of severe premenstrual swelling with large doses of vitamin:

Over the years as I saw more and more patients, oedema (swelling) of the hands during the premenstrual period could be linked with evidence of abdominal distension, involuntary muscle spasms of the legs and feet, and swelling of the eyelids and face. In one group of women I treated for these disorders, four out of eleven of them had previously taken diuretics for control of oedema, with little success. But when they took fifty to one hundred milligrams (mg) of B_6 daily, all their signs and symptoms were relieved[1].

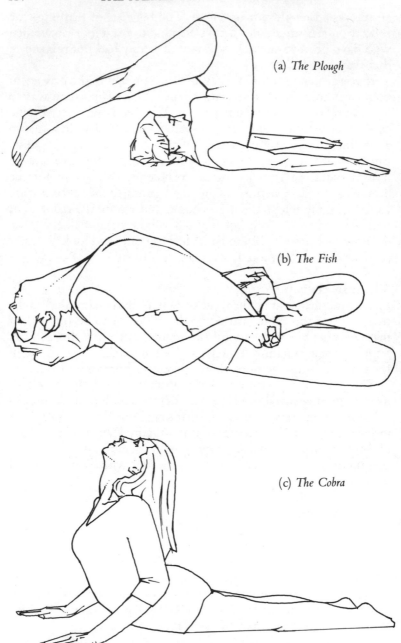

(a) *The Plough*

(b) *The Fish*

(c) *The Cobra*

Figure 4: Yoga Positions

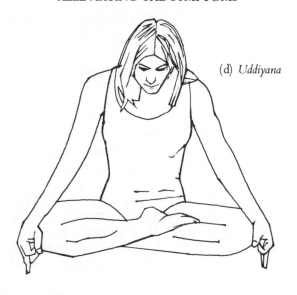

(d) *Uddiyana*

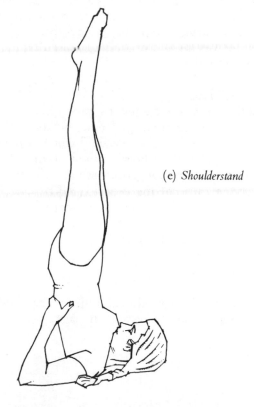

(e) *Shoulderstand*

The usual recommended dose is 40 mg of pyridoxine twice daily, rising to 75 mg twice daily in gradual steps if necessary. It is essential to commence the treatment three days before the expected start of any premenstrual symptoms, in order to derive maximum benefit from it. The tablets can be stopped two to three days after the start of your period. Some doctors recommend taking an extra one or two 20 mg tablets just before the start of the period, since symptoms generally become more severe then. In some clinical trials, patients have required between 100 and 500 mg of pyridoxine every day, to obtain relief from severe symptoms.

Besides taking supplementary supplies of pyridoxine, you may prefer to take this vitamin in a more natural way by including in your diet foods that are rich in it, such as: yeast and liver concentrates; kidney, pork, ham and veal; fresh fish; bananas, avocados, prunes and raisins; peanuts, walnuts and whole-grain cereal.

You can buy tablets of the vitamin from chemists and health-food shops, or ask your doctor for a prescription. Faced with a patient suffering from the premenstrual syndrome, however, many doctors are more likely to prescribe diuretics (water pills) than pyridoxine.

Diuretic drugs
Diuretic drugs are frequently prescribed for women suffering from the premenstrual syndrome, on the grounds that they are capable of mobilizing excess fluid which is being retained by the tissues. The chief criticism aimed at this therapy is that it is symptomatic only and does nothing whatsoever to correct the underlying cause of the waterlogged tissues.

It can be argued, in their favour, that at least diuretics work; and in cases in which the worst symptoms are due to fluid retention, then taking tablets which release the water seems the most straightforward way of handling the trouble. The problem with this defence is that:

(a) diuretics do *not* always relieve the problem (see Ellis's comment[1] on the patients he successfully treated with pyridoxine);

(b) in the words of Dr Katherina Dalton, pioneer in the treatment and diagnosis of women's hormonal illness, in particular the premenstrual syndrome: 'using diuretics is like mopping up the flood on the floor when a pipe bursts, instead of calling the plumber to mend the hole'.

It is about as helpful, in the long-term, as baling out water from the floor of a leaking boat – stop your efforts for a moment and the boat is swamped again. It is true that giving pyridoxine is also a form of symptomatic treatment, and in that sense no better than giving diuretics. But at least in favour of pyridoxine is the fact that when you take it, you are supplementing your diet with a compound that it needs and can utilize in several different essential chemical pathways. You are not just taking a drug whose sole means of helping you is to cause your kidneys to manufacture more urine.

This is what diuretics do. There are several different types of diuretic drugs available, but the simplest of them work by causing the filter tubules of the kidney to get rid of large amounts of mineral salts, in particular potassium chloride. The effect of this is for a correspondingly large volume of water to be excreted together with the salts, which cannot leave the body unless they take a certain minimum amount of water with them. This is the other side of the coin from the effect of taking too much salt in your food. Once it is in the body, and before it can be got rid of, a certain quantity of fluid has to accompany it, and this encourages the storage of water in your tissues rather than encouraging its release in urine.

Another criticism to be fairly levelled at the use of diuretic drugs is that they may cause the body to get rid of excessive amounts of vital salts and minerals – in particular potassium, which is necessary to healthy heart function. So either the patient has to take the diuretics in small quantities, or in addition to taking the diuretic tablets she is also obliged to take a potassium supplement to make good the loss that the diuretic causes. This is why many women prefer to take safe, natural compounds of proven benefit to the body, rather than rely upon drugs which, taken in excess, can harm the bodily systems and sometimes cause other toxic side-effects in addition to potassium deficiency.

Hormone therapy

Approaching the treatment of the premenstrual syndrome by means of artificial hormones is a step in the right direction, because hormonal imbalance is known to play a definite and inseparable role in the production of premenstrual symptoms. It is not, however, the final answer – firstly, because not all women who *should* respond to this treatment in fact do so, and secondly, because it is now known that hormonal upset is an effect of premenstrual disorder, the underlying cause being a deficiency of essential fatty acids (EFAs).

Supplementing the patient with progesterone, in one of its several forms, is based on the supposition that the premenstrual syndrome is caused by a lack of this hormone. When the evidence for this long-accepted theory is scrutinized, there is not a great deal of support for it and progesterone fails to relieve symptoms adequately in most women[2, 3]. When such a deficiency exists, response may be acceptable – but there remains the problem of the side-effects of hormone therapy.

The different forms in which progesterone is available include:

Dydrogesterone
This is closely related to natural progesterone, but with one or two different properties. It is available in tablet form, strength 10 mg, and these are taken twice daily from day twelve until day twenty-six, when the woman's cycle lasts for twenty-eight days. Cycles of different lengths require the timing to be adjusted accordingly. Some women need a slightly higher dose than 20 mg daily.

Natural progesterone
This is available as *Cyclogest* suppositories which contain 200 or 400 mg progesterone. These are generally used for seven to fourteen days premenstrually. The relatively small number of women who use progesterone in this form respond quite satisfactorily to it.

Norethisterone
This is a compound similar to progesterone and is capable of relieving symptoms in some women but the drawback is that side-effects are likely to occur.

Oral contraceptive pill

The Pill helps a number of women suffering from the premenstrual syndrome. It is not thought to be suitable for women over the age of thirty-five years, and although it carries the advantage of acting as a contraceptive method for women wanting to take advantage from this, it is clearly useless when the premenstrual syndrome sufferer wishes to add to her family.

In addition, it is associated with depression, and this seems an unwise choice of therapy since depression is a common feature of the premenstrual syndrome in the first place. Other side-effects associated with the Pill are the occurrence of migraine-type headaches; acute visual disturbances; clotting of the blood, leading to serious conditions such as strokes and thrombophlebitis (clots occurring in a major vein); raised blood pressure and jaundice.

Bromocriptine therapy

As I mentioned in Chapter 5, a few women suffering from the premenstrual syndrome are found to have an excessively high output of the hormone prolactin by their pituitary gland. This is why their hormonal balance gets upset, and they develop symptoms of progesterone deficiency. They respond fairly well to the drug bromocriptine, which cuts down the quantity of prolactin in the blood by suppressing its secretion by the pituitary gland.

But one returns to the original problem when faced with the fact that it is only a few of the many premenstrual syndrome sufferers who ask for help, who have an abnormally high level of this hormone. It is thought that many of the rest may be abnormally sensitive to ordinary levels of it in the blood, due to a lack of essential fatty acids (EFAs). This is one of the effects of a lack of them, and is comparable to their effect upon the body's need for vitamin B_6 (pyridoxine). The pyridoxine level in the blood of a woman suffering premenstrual symptoms may be perfectly normal, but due to a shortage of EFAs the need for it is very greatly increased; 'normal' levels are therefore insufficient, and give the appearance of a deficiency.

For women who have a definite prolactin 'high' demonstrable in their blood, bromocriptine is sometimes prescribed when other medication has failed to give relief. It is regarded as rather a 'last resort' measure because it is a potent drug with several unpleasant side-effects.

Bromocriptine is manufactured under the name *Parlodel*, and can be prescribed either as 2.5 mg tablets, or as 10 mg capsules. Aimed at suppressing the secretion of prolactin by the pituitary gland, the special relief that *Parlodel* can afford is of breast symptoms, but there is also some evidence that it can help headache, mood changes and bloatedness.

It is one of many drugs with more than one type of activity, and you may find it prescribed for elderly people with Parkinson's disease, as well as for premenstrual symptoms. This is not difficult to understand when it is realized that a drug passes through many pathways in the body, before it is finally broken down and excreted in the urine. And it is perfectly possible for it to affect one series of chemical reactions at a certain point of transit, and another series at another point of transit. This is oversimplifying the matter, but you could liken this to a goods train travelling from Euston to Fishguard and delivering, say, mailbags at one station it stops at, crates of milk at another, and all its passengers at yet another.

If *Parlodel* is prescribed for you, you will be introduced to it gradually, going from a low dose to the required amount. This is so that optimum response is achieved with minimum of trouble from side-effects.

With respect to side-effects, there is no doubt that under the circumstances I have outlined, *Parlodel* can give relief from premenstrual symptoms; but as always when a drug is involved one must be chary of the level of toxicity that is bound to accompany its regular administration. Nausea is the commonest side-effect, and dizziness, headache, vomiting, mild constipation and low blood pressure have also been reported.

Tranquillizers
It is a regrettable fact that prescriptions for tranquillizers are still handed out to patients suffering from symptoms of the premenstrual syndrome. This happens when the doctor does not realize that his patient is suffering from this illness, or because in any case he cannot think what else to do for her.

The trouble is that tranquillizers 'help' to relieve intense irritability and a tendency to violent outbursts, but in so doing they 'damp down' a number of functions of the brain, including the centres where emotions are experienced. The result is a feeling of depression – and if you already feel depressed and lethargic, then you are bound to feel much worse.

There is no room at all in the pharmaceutical armament store against the premenstrual syndrome, for tranquillizing drugs. It is an illness with specific causes and specific treatment – and these drugs should not be prescribed even as a 'symptomatic measure' for they are liable to make the overall picture a good deal worse.

If you intend to consult your doctor about premenstrual symptoms, do go to see him *with* the two charts which you have filled in over a period of at least a couple of months. Point out the suggestive timing of your recurrent symptoms and if he suggests a sedative variety of therapy, please ask him for an alternative!

[1] Ellis, J. M. *Vitamin B: The Doctor's Report* (Harper and Row, New York, 1973).

[2] Dalton, K. *The Premenstrual Syndrome* (Heinemann, 1964).

[3] Sampson, G. A. 'The premenstrual syndrome', *British Journal of Psychiatry* 135 (1979), pp.209-215.

10

The Root of the Problem

Recent research has shown that a deficiency of essential fatty acids is the basic defect underlying the premenstrual syndrome. But where do we go from there? What *are* essential fatty acids, why do we need them, and how do we come to lack them? Does a deficiency of them affect the body in any other ways?

To understand what essential fatty acids are, you need to know a fact or two about the structure of fat – a word with which we are all familiar in a variety of contexts, from fashionable shapes and sizes with respect to figure proportions, to the deliciousness of certain animal fats (butter, cream, crackling), to the argument of saturated versus unsaturated fats in the diet. Fats and oils are, chemically speaking, triglycerides, or compounds made from fatty acids neutralized by glycerol (glycerine). The usual fatty acids of dietary fat are oleic, palmitic and stearic and in the body these can be converted to – or synthesized from – acetic acid. Glycerol and acetic acid are both consumed by the same process, incidentally, as sugar to provide energy, and the end-products are the same – water and carbon dioxide.

The only difference between a fat and an oil is consistency. At body temperature human fat is semi-liquid – in fact, it is an oil.

Animal fats solidify at room temperature but their vegetable equivalents remain oily. Several unrelated compounds, for example the lipoids (or lipids), are often classed as fats. Like fats they are insoluble in water and their disposal in the body is closely linked to that of fats. Much the most important of them is one which everyone has heard of, called cholesterol.

Small quantities of fats and lipoids are incorporated into the structure of the body cells and are not available as fuel. They are essential components of the cell walls, and the body would not be able to function without them. The rest of the fat is stored as adipose tissue in various parts of the body, mainly under the skin. We have an excess of it when we are overweight, but in moderation it serves as an insulator and a shock absorber, and can at any time be mobilized as fuel and consumed.

This is what happens when we go on a diet. We limit our calorie intake so that the excess fat under the skin is taken out of the fat store, utilized as fuel to supply energy and weight is lost. Or we step up our exercise so that more fuel is needed than is provided by what we eat, and again the fat is mobilized and weight is lost. Fats and lipoids can be synthesized in the body from carbohydrates and so should not be essential to the diet. But they are a convenient food, for a small quantity provides much energy – weight for weight, twice as much as protein or carbohydrate – and fat is eaten more or less pure, without the large amount of water that goes into the cooking of starchy food. A diet without any fat in it has to be extremely bulky to provide enough energy, but beyond the convenience issue there is no doubt that some fat is necessary for good health.

Besides other things, a diet short of fat often lacks the fat-soluble vitamins A and D and it is also very unpalatable. But there is more to the story than that: the actual quality of fat affects health. If some 'essential' fatty acids are lacking, then excessive amounts of cholesterol accumulate and damage arteries. These essential acids are found in vegetable oils and, to a far lesser extent, in animal fats.

Essential fatty acids can be compared to vitamins. They are sometimes known as vitamin F, and are substances which cannot be made by the body but must be taken in with food. They were discovered at the University of Minnesota by George and Mildred

Burr, in 1930, and these two workers found that all animals and humans need to include them in their diets. This has been confirmed by all the subsequent work done on these substances.

In animals who are totally deprived of essential fatty acids (EFAs), many serious problems develop. They cannot resist infection; they have very bad skin and their hair falls out; fibrous tissue and other substances that keeps cells in a coherent mass do not form properly; they become infertile; they develop painful, swollen joints; their livers become damaged; and they become lethargic and irritable.

By far the most important EFA is linoleic acid. The Burrs and others found that, in most animals, *linoleic acid alone could correct all these problems!*

You may wonder why there has been relatively little interest in essential fatty acid deficiency until recently. Diseases resembling those caused by EFA deficiency, such as the ones mentioned above, are common, but the reason that no one seriously considered the possibility that a lack of EFAs might be involved in these problems, is that the animal studies indicate that an actual deficiency is unlikely. They show that if about one per cent of the total calorie intake is taken in the form of EFAs then all the signs of deficiency are corrected.

Very few human diets indeed contain less than one per cent of the total calories as linoleic acid, and so few people had ever considered the possibility that essential fatty acid deficiency might be common. But there is a major flaw in this reasoning, as was recently revealed.

Oddly enough, although few people have believed that such a deficiency could cause human disease, essential fatty acids are the one vital nutrient which is recommended by the medical profession to be taken in mega doses. For essential fatty acids go under another name – they are polyunsaturates.[1] When doctors recommend people to increase their 'polyunsaturate' intake – in order to lower the amount of cholesterol in the blood, to lower blood pressure and body weight, and to reduce the risk of having heart attacks and strokes – the one active component of the diet is linoleic acid.

Authoritative committee after committee in country after country has recommended that polyunsaturate (essential fatty acid) intake should be far above the minimum one per cent of total calorie intake. Ten per cent is commonly recommended, and most suggest fifteen to twenty per cent. These really are mega doses of an essential nutrient and they have received almost unanimous medical approval.

The flaw in the reasoning is apparent when we see what happens to linoleic acid when it gets into our bodies. Linoleic acid itself is almost inert as an essential fatty acid and it is useless unless it can be activated, and converted into substances of vital importance biochemically to us. In other words, linoleic acid is necessary – but only because it is the starter substance from which active ingredients can be made.

The way in which this comes about involves a series of chemical reactions, starting with linoleic acid and ending with the finished product which is one of a group of substances called prostaglandins, about which more later. You can see the stages of conversion from raw substance (linoleic acid) to final product (prostaglandin) in Figure 5. The first step is the conversion of linoleic acid into a substance known for short as GLA (gammalinolenic acid).

Figure 5: Pathway of metabolism

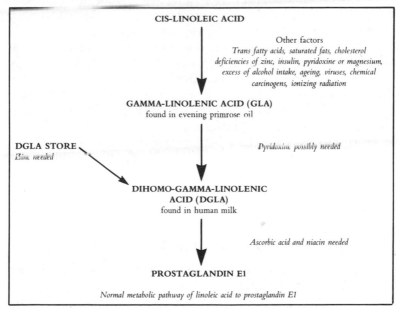

CIS-LINOLEIC ACID

Other factors
Trans fatty acids, saturated fats, cholesterol deficiencies of zinc, insulin, pyridoxine or magnesium, excess of alcohol intake, ageing, viruses, chemical carcinogens, ionizing radiation

GAMMA-LINOLENIC ACID (GLA)
found in evening primrose oil

DGLA STORE
Zinc needed

Pyridoxine possibly needed

DIHOMO-GAMMA-LINOLENIC ACID (DGLA)
found in human milk

Ascorbic acid and niacin needed

PROSTAGLANDIN E1

Normal metabolic pathway of linoleic acid to prostaglandin E1

Regardless of the quantity of linoleic acid present in the diet, if it cannot be converted to GLA it is unable to be of use to us. The most exciting nutritional development over the last fifteen years has been the discovery that a large number of factors block the formation of GLA, thus rendering the dietary linoleic acid almost useless. The work was pioneered by Rodolfo Brenner, in Argentina, and has since been substantiated by many laboratories and universities in the USA, Canada, the United Kingdom and Europe. Moreover, it has been discovered that only one form of linoleic acid, called in chemical jargon its 'cis' form, is capable of being converted into GLA. Cis-linoleic acid is found in many vegetables, and particularly in vegetable oils. But, unfortunately, when such oils are heated, deodorized, hydrogenated or otherwise artificially processed, much of the natural, useful linoleic acid is converted into the 'trans' form. This is not an essential fatty acid and it cannot function in the same beneficial way as cis-linoleic acid because it is incapable of being converted into GLA.

In fact, trans-linoleic acid is worse than useless because it has an anti-vitamin effect on the useful cis form, and when it is present it prevents the latter from undergoing the conversion it would normally experience. Yet all the estimates of linoleic acid intake, are of 'total' linoleic acid content, lumping together cis (useful) with trans (useless) forms of this substance, assuming that they are equally valuable. This of course is nonsense. As a result, the actual intake of linoleic acid in its active, useful form has been grossly overestimated in many countries. Since trans acids are abundant in most margarines, the majority of people who think that they are increasing their intake of valuable polyunsaturates by eating this in the place of butter, are probably doing nothing of the kind.

What factors other than the presence of 'anti-vitamin' trans-linoleic acid, block the vital formation of GLA? Our list of the factors capable of this is almost certainly incomplete, but the ones we know about already make interesting reading. The known causes of inadequate GLA formation include:

(a) the presence of trans-linoleic acid (see above);

(b) a diet rich in saturated fats, such as that eaten in the UK, the USA and similar cultures;

(c) diabetes;

(d) the moderate to high consumption of alcohol – this refers not only to alcoholics but also to about twenty per cent of the adult population, who are probably consuming sufficient alcohol to interfere with GLA formation;

(e) the ageing process; there is a great deal of current interest in the idea that a loss of the ability to make GLA may be one of the most significant factors in ageing;

(f) insufficient zinc, magnesium and vitamin B_6 (pyridoxine), all of which are necessary to GLA formation;

(g) viral infections, radiation and cancer.

The list is impressive. Many people in this country are exposed to one or several of the factors that block GLA formation and this of course affects the two sexes equally. In the presence of these factors, the formation of GLA from linoleic acid may be very severely restricted. It is possible that the medical profession and expert nutritionists are forced to recommend mega doses of essential fatty acids since only then can enough GLA be formed, to protect against diseases of the heart and the circulation.

What about the stages following GLA formation, on the way to producing the prostaglandin substances? Most of the GLA (see Figure 5) is rapidly converted into DGLA (dihomogammalinolenic acid). This is capable of being converted to a number of compounds, the most important of which is PGE 1 (prostaglandin), so called because it belongs to the E1 series of this substance. In addition to GLA, PGE 1 is another name which will become a household word within the next ten years. Leading laboratories in many countries have shown that it has a range of vital and desirable actions, far and away more complex and numerous than was at first suspected.

The prostaglandins themselves constitute a group of substances, all of which are derived from fatty acids, which were initially identified in 1935 when they were thought to originate in the prostate gland. They are now known to occur in most tissues, and to have various biological actions which may mimic hormonal activity. The 'vital and desirable actions' of prostaglandin E1, mentioned above, include the following:

(a) it prevents thrombosis and lowers the blood pressure;

(b) it opens up blood vessels and relieves angina;

(c) it slows down the speed with which cholesterol is made;

(d) it enables insulin to work more efficiently;

(e) it prevents inflammation and controls arthritis;

(f) it has many different actions on the brain, and in humans it produces a sense of well-being;

(g) under laboratory conditions it stops cancer cells from growing;

(h) it relieves the physical and mental symptoms of the premenstrual syndrome.

There is very little doubt that the many desirable actions of essential fatty acids depend upon their conversion within the body along the chemical pathway we have looked at, i.e. into GLA, DGLA and PGE 1.

Clearly, with such problems existing with respect to the availability of cis-linoleic acid and its subsequent conversion into GLA, it is natural to question whether GLA or DGLA are ever found naturally occurring in foods. Both of these substances are found in tiny amounts in a wide variety of foods, but only two food sources contain them in substantial amounts. Both GLA and DGLA are found in human milk – breast-fed infants in their first year consume 50-250 mg of GLA and DGLA every day. Cow's milk contains no GLA and only about one quarter of the DGLA present in human milk. This is one of the many reasons why breast milk is a great deal better for babies than cow's milk.

The only other substantial source of GLA is the seed oil of a plant known as the Evening Primrose. This plant originated in the east of the United States and was extensively used by American Indians for medical purposes. Extracts of the whole plant were believed to have healing properties when applied to wounds and to inflamed skin. Taken internally, the plant was thought to hasten recovery from infections and to be of particular value to patients with asthma.

The Evening Primrose was one of the first plants to be exported to Europe, where it acquired the common name of King's Cure-all. Modern research has confirmed its value in asthma and has demonstrated that it has a range of properties that would have astonished the ancient herbalists. The wild plant has now been domesticated and its oil-bearing properties greatly improved by breeding methods. The best quality oil now contains about nine per cent by weight of GLA, and the remaining ninety-one per cent is very similar to safflower or sunflower oil, containing seventy-two per cent of cis-linoleic acid.

The pure unprocessed oil is available in plain gelatin capsules containing 250 or 500 mg of the oil, together with safflower and linseed oil to make up bulk and contribute to the total quantity of cis-linoleic acid. The GLA is kept in optimum condition by the addition of pure vitamin E. Two to four of the 500 mg capsules contain about as much GLA as the DGLA found in human milk and consumed daily by a baby in the first year of its life. GLA is very rapidly converted to DGLA in the body, and the two are nutritionally equivalent.

The above capsule content specifications apply only to the Evening Primrose oil sold under the name of *Efamol* – the oil on which all the world-wide clinical trials have been carried out. We shall look more closely at *Efamol* and how it should be used, below.

You may wonder *why* GLA and DGLA are found in human milk. The short answer is that we do not yet know – but it is possible to make some intelligent guesses. Brenner has found in animals that the ability to form GLA does not develop until after birth. The development of human infants is in many respects delayed compared to that of the young of other species – and it is very possible that the ability of some human infants to form GLA and thereby DGLA could be considerably delayed. So in order to cater for this, the GLA and the DGLA could be secreted directly into the milk of the mother, to be immediately available to the young infant.

Recent research has shown that prostaglandin E1, and therefore DGLA, are necessary to cells in the bloodstream called T suppressor lymphocytes, essential for preventing the development of eczema and allergies. The well-known fact that allergies and

eczema are more common in bottle- than in breast-fed babies, can
perhaps be explained by a relative lack of DGLA in the bottle-fed
children. Certainly this is born out by observation. Babies who
develop eczema on changing from breast- to bottle-feeding, are
generally dramatically healed by rubbing into their unaffected
skin 500-1000 mg of *Efamol* morning and evening. This contains
about as much GLA as the daily DGLA intake from breast milk,
and when the oil is rubbed into unaffected areas of skin it is
absorbed just as effectively as it is by swallowing.

Evening Primrose oil is currently being studied in top
laboratories all over the world and experiments with animals
shows it to have some highly desirable effects, in addition to those
listed as properties of PGE 1 earlier in this chapter. It can slow
down the rate of growth of experimental breast cancer, reduce
body weight in obese mice and its effect on cats is worth
mentioning too. Cats cannot make GLA from linoleic acid – they
have something wrong with their chemistry similar to the defect in
human chemistry that prevents us from making vitamin C. Just
as we have become adapted to this by using much less vitamin C
per day than those animals which make it for themselves, so cats
have 'learned' to manage with very little GLA or DGLA. This
probably explains their liking for milk, for although cow's milk
contains very little DGLA compared to human milk, it contains a
lot compared to other foods. When cats are fed a diet containing
only linoleic acid as a source of fat, they develop all the problems
that other animals get when linoleic acid is excluded from the diet.
Their skin condition becomes very poor, their fur falls out, they
become highly susceptible to infection, they suffer from liver
damage and they become infertile. Evening Primrose oil containing
GLA has a dramatic effect on correcting these problems. In
Siamese cats, which seem especially susceptible to skin disease,
adding Evening Primrose oil to their food quickly produces
complete healing.

Extensive laboratory studies on essential fatty acids and PGE 1,
and a broad acceptance of the need for a high polyunsaturate
intake to control diseases of the heart and circulation, have
stimulated many investigators to study the effect of the 'super'
polyunsaturate Evening Primrose oil. In theory, large amounts of
this oil should have the same effect as much larger quantities of

other oils because the GLA in it bypasses the blockages in GLA formation. In some people in whom, for one reason or another, GLA cannot be formed, the oil should have effects which cannot be achieved by other polyunsaturate sources, no matter what vast quantities are consumed.

This theory has been borne out in practice and Evening Primrose oil has been found to have the following effects when taken in amounts of 2-4 g per day (four to eight capsules), with half taken in the morning and half in the evening:

(a) it lowers blood cholesterol levels as effectively as drugs;

(b) it lowers blood pressure (hypertension) to normal;

(c) it did not affect the weight of people whose weight was normal, but over half of those who were obese lost weight, even though they made no attempt to alter their eating habits;[1]

(d) it improves eczema in both children and adults and in some instances it produces complete healing;[2]

(e) in about two thirds of patients with mild to moderate arthritis it stopped the disease process completely – interestingly, most of those who got better felt transiently worse about two weeks after starting the course and then improved;[3]

(f) it clears up many cases of 'dry eyes' and 'dry mouth' in people who do not produce enough tears or saliva, especially when given in conjunction with pyridoxine and vitamin C;[4]

(g) it clears up soft, brittle, flaky nails after three to four weeks;[5]

(h) it alleviates hangovers and the depression that follows heavy drinking;[6]

(i) it has dramatic effects in children suffering from hyperactivity which according to research performed by the HCSG (the Hyperactive Children's Support Group) seems to be due to a deficiency of essential fatty acids;[7]

(j) in this country, the patients' pressure group ARMS (Action through Research into Multiple Sclerosis) has accumulated evidence to suggest that Evening Primrose oil slows down the progression of the disease – this is naturally highly controversial but ARMS is willing to give its evidence to any enquirers[8, 9];

(k) given with zinc, Evening Primrose oil produces remarkable results in many cases of acne;

(l) finally, and most relevantly – **women taking Evening Primrose oil for other reasons reported some time ago dramatic relief from the premenstrual syndrome.** The Evening Primrose oil relieved physical and mental symptoms and these reports have been confirmed by studies at major centres for premenstrual studies.

Before we look at how exactly the premenstrual syndrome is helped by *Efamol*, it must be mentioned that a number of nutrients are known to be important to the efficient use of essential fatty acids by the body. Included are magnesium and pyridoxine, vitamin B_3 (niacin or nitocinamide) vitamin E and selenium. The two of particular interest are zinc and Vitamin C, since research during the last three years has shown that they are necessary for the formation of prostaglandin E1 from DGLA, the last stage in the chemical synthetic chain. There is now plenty of evidence that PGE 1 formation is crucial to the actions of both these nutrients. Furthermore, the effects of both zinc and vitamin C may be very greatly diminished if supplies of GLA and DGLA are inadequate. It is now possible to make the following statement:

The premenstrual syndrome is due, entirely or largely, to a deficiency of essential fatty acids. This deficiency is not due only to a lack of the active fatty acid, i.e. cis-linoleic acid, in the diet. It is due also to the blockages that occur in the utilization of available acid to form the vital substances of which it is the ground substance. There are also a number of factors responsible for the blocking effect: a prominent one is the presence of linoleic acid in its 'anti-vitamin' or trans form. This is formed from active, naturally occurring cis-linoleic acid by the industrial processes to which the latter is subjected during the refining processes, and also in cooking when it is subjected to high temperatures, for example, during prolonged deep-fat frying. It prevents the conversion of cis-linoleic acid into GLA.

Because of the blocking factors that interfere with this conversion, a great deal of the linoleic acid in our diets is failing to act as a source of essential fatty acids as was always supposed, and very few polyunsaturate diets are likely to achieve their intended goal.

The end-product PGE 1 is necessary for hormonal balance during the premenstrual syndrome and a lack of it produces the symptoms of the premenstrual syndrome. One of the best ways of overcoming the essential fatty acid deficiency causing premenstrual symptoms and a wide variety of other complaints, is to bypass the conversion stage at which blocking occurs by providing the individual with pure GLA.

Two substances contain this in appreciable amounts – one is human breast milk and the other is the oil from the seeds of the Evening Primrose flower. *Efamol* is the form of the oil which has been used in all the research, investigations and clinical trials into the properties of this substance, and is stabilized by means of the added nutrient vitamin E.

[1] Vaddadi, K. S. and Horrobin, D. F. 'Weight loss produced by evening primrose oil administration in normal and schitzophrenic individuals', *IRCS Journal of Medical Science* 7 (1979), p.52.

[2] Lovell, C. R., Burton, J. L. and Horrobin, D. F. 'Treatment of atopic eczema with evening primrose oil', *Lancet* 1 (1981), p.278.

[3] McCormick, J. N., Neill, W. A. and Sim, A. K. 'Immunosuppressive effect of linoleic acid', *Lancet* 2 (1977), p.508.

[4] Horrobin, D. F. and Campbell, A. C. 'Sjofren's syndrome and the sicca syndrome: the role of prostaglandin E1 deficiency', *Medical Hypotheses* 6 (1980), pp. 255-232.

[5] Campbell, A. C. and MacEwan, G. C. 'Treatment of brittle nails and dry eyes', *British Journal of Dermatology* (1983).

[6] Lieb, J. Dept. of Psychiatry, Yale University, USA. Personal communication (1980).

[7] Colquhoun, V. and Bunday, S. 'A lack of essential fatty acids as a possible cause of hyperactivity in children', *Medical Hypotheses* 7 (1980), pp.681-686.

[8] Swank, R. L. 'Multiple sclerosis: twenty years on a low fat diet', *Archives of Neurology* 23 (1970), p.460.

[9] Swank, R. L. *The Multiple Sclerosis Diet Book* (Doubleday, New York, 1977).

11

The Modern Solution

The reason why so many systems, including the female reproductive system, are affected adversely by a deficiency of essential fatty acids, is because the end-products of their metabolism, prosta-glandin E1 series, are vital chemicals that play essential roles in many different biochemical systems in the body.

The name of 'Cure-all', if coined nowadays, would probably have a derisory ring, especially if a particular substance were claimed to heal a wide variety of ills, from colds on the chest to warts – not forgetting its powers of restoring the hair and keeping the bowels regular. This array of abilities reminds one of some of the patent medicines much favoured by small-ads readers earlier this century, and which had as their chief claim to efficacy the ability to make money on behalf of their perpetrators!

When many different claims are made on behalf of one product, particularly when its target areas appear to be highly divergent, the herb, drug or plant extract immediately comes under suspicion, and a common situation is that it is marketed by charlatans and bought by fools. When the name 'King's Cure-all', however, was adopted for the Evening Primrose flower, it was a serious name resulting from the considered opinion of experienced herbalists and physicians, who discovered to their amazement and gratification the effective uses to which preparations of the herb could be put.

If the plant had been dubbed 'Poor Man's Cure-all' it would have been a little less impressive. But 'King's Cure-all' tells us that the plant was considered worthy to treat the ailments of the monarch himself. It is because the oil from its seeds contains the vital GLA in considerable quantities and obviates the need for any other attempts to overcome the harmful blockages, that the drug can be so widely effective. So it is now true that nutritional approaches can give dramatic relief to sufferers of the premenstrual syndrome.

As we have seen, most women with the premenstrual syndrome have normal prolactin levels, but their body tissues may be abnormally sensitive to normal levels of this hormone when essential fatty acids – and therefore prostaglandin E1 – are deficient. It is in this way that an EFA deficiency can lead to an apparent excess of prolactin, and symptoms related to a progesterone and oestrogen imbalance can be produced. We have also seen that pyridoxine can be effective in the premenstrual syndrome, and that pyridoxine increases the efficiency with which EFAs are used by the body. This helps to explain the successful treatment of a number of symptoms with pyridoxine.

Regarding trials of essential fatty acids in the premenstrual syndrome, one of the largest and most experienced premenstrual syndrome clinics in the world, at St Thomas' Hospital, London, has been involved closely with these studies. Dr Michael Brush has just completed a study of *Efamol* treatment in over seventy women who had failed to respond to one, and in many cases two, other types of treatment.

Efamol is the form of the oil of the Evening Primrose flower to have been used in clinical trial work, as it is pure, stable and reliable. It has therefore been subjected to rigorous clinical testing and all the claims made on its behalf have been put forward only after the proof has been available to substantiate them.

A carefully controlled clinical study into the effects of *Efamol* on breast pain was carried out at the Universities of Wales and Dundee in one hundred women.[1] In many of these women the pain became much worse premenstrually. This study showed a highly significant effect of *Efamol* in relieving breast pain.

In the trial conducted at St Thomas' hospital, sixty-eight women with severe premenstrual symptoms in whom standard forms of treatment had failed, were treated with *Efamol*, two 500 mg capsules twice daily after food. Some of the worst received continuous treatment but most started treatment three days before the expected start of symptoms. A few of the worst patients received three capsules twice daily, and some, too, were given pyridoxine either alone or in the mineral/vitamin compound *Efavite*, concurrently with *Efamol*. The women who received pyridoxine were known to have obtained insufficient relief from pyridoxine given as sole treatment.[2]

Endocrine and other biochemical conditions were eliminated by measuring the women's basic hormonal profiles; these included serum prolactin, FSH, LH, progesterone and plasma oestradiol. Other biochemical tests were carried out if indicated, to make sure there was no unknown malfunction causing lack of response to standard treatment.

Details of the patients – their ages and previous forms of treatment – are as follows:

Efamol and Premenstrual Syndrome

Age Range: 21-48 years

Previous treatments (partial success in some cases):

Diuretics	(15)	Dydrogesterone	(19)
Psychotropics	(23)	Pyridoxine	(58)
Progesterone	(12)	O.C's	(14)
Norethisterone	(9)	Others	(18)

Very marked improvement was seen in sixty-one per cent of patients and twenty-three per cent showed partial relief. Fifteen per cent showed no significant change. The full range of premenstrual syndrome symptoms was improved, including depression, anxiety, irritability, headache, breast discomfort and fluid retention. Thirty-six patients complained of very painful breasts (mastodynia) and of these twenty-six reported good relief, five reported moderate relief and five, no help. Side-effects were limited to minor skin blemishes in three patients and 'damping down' of mood in another three. Of nine patients suffering from fibrocystic breasts, six reported good response, while three had no response.

Here are details of four of the women taking part in this trial.

Case 1

Marian B was a twenty-six-year-old domestic manager who had never been pregnant but who complained of symptoms clearly suggesting the premenstrual syndrome for ten to fourteen days before each period, over the previous six years.

Her cycles were twenty-nine days long and her main complaints were of severe breast discomfort, irritability, tearfulness, poor co-ordination and diminished concentration. She had had no relief from dydrogesterone, norethisterone or progesterone suppositories. Pyridoxine had given relief at first (75 mg twice daily) but this had not lasted. There were no abnormal blood levels.

She was given *Efamol* 500 mg, two capsules twice daily from day seven to the start of the period, in addition to pyridoxine. This proved very useful, although the breast discomfort continued.

When the *Efamol* was increased to three capsules twice daily plus six *Efavite* capsules, breast discomfort was eliminated.

Case 2

Fay D was a forty-year-old school helper who had attended the premenstrual syndrome clinic several times during the previous four years. Her complaints consisted of irritability, anxiety, depression, poor co-ordination, loss of libido and moderate fluid retention but no breast discomfort. Her blood levels showed no abnormalities.

Past treatment had consisted of dydrogesterone and the anti-depressant drug tranylcypromine, neither of which had helped. Pyridoxine, 75 mg twice daily, had helped only slightly. When she was given *Efamol*, two capsules twice daily, and *Efavite*, one capsule twice daily, together with pyridoxine, 100 mg daily, her symptoms disappeared and have never returned.

Case 3

Rosalind M was a thirty-four-year-old school secretary and had been suffering from premenstrual syndrome for five years. These had been worse since sterilization two years previously, which she had had despite the fact that she had never had any pregnancies. Her symptoms were severe breast pain, swelling of the abdomen and the face, depression and irritability which lasted for the last fourteen days of her twenty-eight to twenty-nine day cycle.

She had been treated with tranquillizers, pyridoxine and diuretics and had obtained no relief from any of them. Investigations showed no abnormality, with respect to blood levels, of prolactin and oestradiol. She was started on four capsules of *Efamol* daily and 80 ml of pyridoxine twice daily. This produced very great improvement in mood – and some improvement in swelling and in breast discomfort, all of which were maintained for as long as the patient was seen at the clinic.

Case 4
Jacqueline O was a thirty-four-year-old housewife with a history of two pregnancies and one live birth. She had had symptoms of the premenstrual syndrome for the previous eight years. These consisted of lethargy, mood swings (depression, irritability), troublesome bloating, very painful breasts, and bad co-ordination for the fourteen days prior to her period starting in a twenty-eight day cycle.

She had received no benefit from the diuretics, progesterone suppositories and pyridoxine 40 mg daily, which had been prescribed for her. Laboratory investigations were normal, and she was started on four capsules of *Efamol* daily, plus four tablets of *Efavite* daily. These gave complete relief.

An overview of the clinical trials and research into the use of *Efamol* in the premenstrual syndrome suggests that it is of help to nine out of ten women with premenstrual symptoms. So it has a very high success rate, even when compared with long-established traditional treatment such as we have discussed.

The two other major points in its favour are, firstly, that it corrects the underlying essential fatty acid deficiency at source by supplying what the body needs, thereby reaching to the root of the problem. It is not 'symptomatic' therapy, as it approaches the problem with a view to eradicating it rather than simply seeking to allay its unpleasant signs. Secondly, being a natural food product and not a synthetic drug, it is completely non-toxic and safe to use.

Recent studies suggest that the following is the best way of using *Efamol* for premenstrual illness: take two 500mg capsules of *Efamol* (together with *Efavite*) three times a day throughout the menstrual cycle, dropping to one capsule two or three times a day after two months. Extra pyridoxine may be added to this, in a dose of 50mg twice per day, during the fourteen days before menstruation is expected.

*   *   *   *

I hope you have found this book useful. I started to treat patients suffering from the premenstrual syndrome with *Efamol* in 1981 – or rather told them about it and suggested that they buy it from either a health-food shop or chemist, since it was not then available on prescription. Each of my patients who has tried *Efamol* for premenstrual illness has gained some relief, and more than ninety per cent of them have had total relief.

I hope that the combination of *Efamol* and this book will succeed in their joint objective of helping to eliminate the premenstrual syndrome.

[1] Pashby, N. L., Mansel, R. R., Preece, P. E., Hughes, L. E. and Aspinall, J. 'A clinical trial of evening primrose oil *(Efamol)* in mastalgia'. Paper given at a meeting of the British Surgical Research Society, Cardiff (July 1981).

[2] Brush, M. G. and Taylor, R. W. 'Gammalinolenic acid *(Efamol)* in the treatment of premenstrual syndrome'.

Index

Other titles in this series...

COMING LATE TO MOTHERHOOD
Joan Michelson and Sue Gee

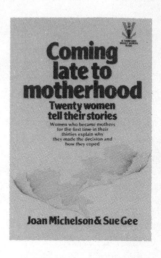

An increasing number of women now postpone having their first child, and the purpose of this book is to dispel or support some of the general notions which surround women becoming mothers for the first time in their thirties. This achieved by a compilation of other women's experiences with particular reference to their reactions to the abrupt change to their lifestyle that the transition to motherhood brings, so that support and guidance can be drawn from knowing how others coped.

SEX DURING PREGNANCY AND AFTER CHILDBIRTH
Sylvia Close SANC

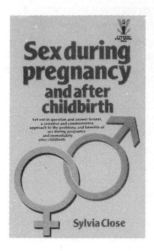

Pregnancy and the weeks immediately after childbirth pose particular problems to a sexual relationship, and it is the author's experience over many years as an ante-natal teacher that people are not always aware of or prepared for some of these problems. This book deals with the subject in a question and answer style, and the author puts across both sound advice and reassurance for young couples.